NEVER BE
TIRED AGAIN!

NEVER BE TIRED AGAIN!

DR. DAVID C. GARDNER
DR. GRACE JOELY BEATTY

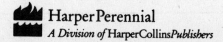
HarperPerennial
A Division of HarperCollinsPublishers

For information on Never Be Tired Again workshops, seminars, in-house training and the newsletter, please contact Swandigo Marketing and Promotion, P.O. Box 1786, Pacific Palisades, CA 90272-1786.

A hardcover edition of this book was originally published in 1988 by Rawson Associates. It is here reprinted by arrangement with Rawson Associates.

First PERENNIAL LIBRARY edition published 1990.

Library of Congress Cataloging-in-Publication Data

Gardner, David C., 1934–
Never be tired again / David C. Gardner, Grace Joely Beatty.—
1st Perennial Library ed.
p. cm.
Includes bibliographical references.
ISBN 0-06-097298-X
1. Health. 2. Vitality. 3. Fatigue—Prevention. Nutrition.
5. Exercise. I. Beatty, Grace Joely, 1947–. II. Title.
RA776.5.G373 1990 90-6749
613.7—dc20

01 00 99 98 RRD(H) 20 19

For our parents, Jessica and Raymond, Shirley and Joseph, who gave us a love of learning and taught us that books are special treasures

Contents

Acknowledgments

Authors like to think of themselves as independent. However, every author is actually dependent upon many people. We are no different. We would like gratefully to acknowledge the support, encouragement, and assistance of the following:

Norman Lobsenz, for his outstanding editorial assistance. He was supportive and professional and at all times the perfect editor. The end result was that not only our book but our lives were enriched by our association with him.

Bill Gladstone, our agent, who encouraged us to go ahead with the project and who spent endless time making it all happen.

Eleanor Rawson, our publisher, for her excellent suggestions, criticisms, and ideas that ultimately made this book a reality.

Grace Shaw, our managing editor, for her insightful and supportive fine tuning.

Chef Daniel Bumgardner, for lending his considerable culinary skills in helping us develop the healthy gourmet recipes for this book.

Joseph and Shirley Beatty, for their love and emotional support, as well as for countless hours of reading and feedback sessions.

Jessica Gardner and Joshua Gardner, who understood when Daddy and Joely had to write rather than play.

Paula Gardner and David Capaldo, for their understanding and support.

Asher Schapiro, for always being there for us from day one.

David Sauer, of Boston University, for his assistance in helping to keep us up to date on the research in nutrition, medicine, psychology, and physics that forms the scientific foundation for this book.

Bob and Lorraine Dyson, who arranged a very special kind of support that freed us up to concentrate on writing.

Andrea Davis, for her incredible computer and word processing assistance.

Sioux Ackerman, for her continuous support and for keeping the books straight.

Micki Truman and "KJ" Kjeldahl, of 48 Hour Software, Carlsbad, California, for helping us convert to "state-of-the art" technology in record time. Without their support, we would still be trying to unscramble overloaded floppies.

We want additionally to acknowledge the helpful feedback and suggestions from Sharon Beatty-Parsons; Paul Beatty-Parsons; Ray Bumgardner, J.D.; Carole Bumgardner; Carola Eastwood; Jeremy Geffen, M.D.; Cynthia Gladstone; Salim Nurani, M.D.; Michael Spatuzzi, M.A., Lic. Ac.; John Whitaker, Ph.D.; Linda Whitaker, Ph.D.; and Penelope Young, L.C.S.W.

Last but not least we want to acknowledge the love, support, and personal involvement of all our clients, patients, and friends in the development and refinement of the *Never Be Tired Again!* program.

Part I

THE NEVER BE TIRED AGAIN PROGRAM

Chapter 1

What This Book Can Do for You

Are you sick and tired of being tired? Have you ever prayed, "God, if I can just lie down for an hour I promise I'll get everything done tomorrow"?

You are not alone. Chronic exhaustion is one of the most common complaints medical doctors, counselors, and psychotherapists hear from their patients. But chronic exhaustion is rarely the result of illness or depression, or even just lack of sleep. It is most often the result of poor body chemistry, an energy-draining lifestyle, and psychological stress.

This book will change all that.

This book shows you how to have more energy than you ever dreamed possible. It will help you to develop the extra supply of energy to do and accomplish all the things you've always *wanted* to do, but couldn't because you were too tired from doing all the things you *must* do.

This book teaches you how to create energy to protect yourself against disease, to heal yourself, to work, to play—energy to spare. If you follow our Never Be Tired Again program for just one week, you will notice an incredible increase in your energy level. If you stay on our program, you can expect not only to increase your energy level beyond your wildest dreams but also to:

- Lose fat weight (as opposed to water weight or lean muscle tissue)
- Lower your cholesterol level
- Lower your blood pressure
- Decrease your risk of heart problems, cancer, and other lifestyle-associated diseases

You can expect even more. Here's what some of the people who have successfully completed our Never Be Tired Again program have to say about it.

I spent one year on the program of a prominent New York heart specialist and gained one pound. He told me my cholesterol problem was genetic and my cholesterol count would never dip below 220. In seven days on *your* program my cholesterol dropped from 260 to the safe zone of 182. In seven days I lost six pounds! In seven days I was able to stop taking my allergy medication for the first time in twenty years. I can't believe the incredible energy that comes from living your lifestyle.

> Chief executive officer,
> National employment benefits provider

I lost thirty-five pounds in four months. I've never had so much energy. I look and feel years younger. And the great thing about it is that your program is easy to follow and easy to stick with!

> Chief executive officer,
> Real estate holding company
> Chairman, a major league sports team

Your program is fantastic. I've never had so much energy. When I came to you, I would rate my energy level as a "2." It is now an "8" and climbing. I've been told I look twenty years younger and I certainly feel it. I've lost twenty pounds in two months.

> Senior vice-president,
> National financial analysis firm

My energy level is incredible since I've taken your program. Not only that, I've lost twenty-five pounds in six months and have regained my figure. Something very special happens to people in your program.

> President,
> Fashion industry supplier

PROVEN BENEFITS OF THE "NEVER BE TIRED AGAIN!" PROGRAM

During the past five years our Never Be Tired Again program has been tested on hundreds of people in our one- and two-day seminar series, in our private practice, and, more recently, during a year of intensive research in 1986–87 with forty-one clients participating in our eight-day live-in program. Blood tests were made at the start and end of the program. We found that in seven days clients

- *Reduced their cholesterol* levels an average of 15 percent, with some individuals reducing their levels as much as 34 percent. Follow-up studies show that for those who began our program with dangerously high cholesterol levels (over 250), continuing the program on their own brought 95 percent of them into the minimum risk zone (a level of less than 180) in about five months.
- *Reduced their triglycerides* (fat in the bloodstream) by an average of 35 percent, with some people dropping more than 100 points.
- *Showed an average weight loss of six pounds* (range: five to ten pounds) with continuing weight losses of up to thirty-five pounds in just five months. Subsequent testing showed that for the most part the lost weight constituted fat, not water or muscle tissue.
- *Reduced their blood pressure.* For those on blood pressure medication, the medication was either eliminated or reduced at the end of the seven-day period.
- *Reduced their overall body measurements an average of four inches,* with a special few losing an incredible twelve inches overall in just one week. Overall body measurements are calculated by summing up the girths of the upper arms, chest, waist, hips, and thighs.
- *Rated their energy level as "dramatically" increased.* In follow-up studies, reports of increased energy and productivity are almost unanimous.

WHAT MAKES THE NEVER BE TIRED AGAIN PROGRAM DIFFERENT?

We know that this program works. The people who have been in our program are living proof that it works. However, as someone who has bought this book, you are entitled to ask us *how* we know it works.

That's a good question, because many books today claim you can change your life if you do what they tell you to do. Some of these books contain good advice, some offer eccentric advice, and some offer advice that has been called downright dangerous. They all have one thing in common, however: They talk about only *one part* of your life.

As a human being you are more than the food you eat and the air you breathe. You are more than the way you exercise. You are more than muscles, blood, and bone. You are more than your electromagnetic fields. You are more than your thought waves. We found in our research that *all* of these facets of the real you are important. All of them need to be discussed, because they are all connected. This book brings them all together, shows you how they are connected, and then teaches you how to use that knowledge to your advantage. It is a case of synergy: the whole being greater than the sum of the parts. Is is the human energy dynamic.

This book has no crazy theories we want to test on you. We know each of the elements of our program works by itself because each piece is based on solid scientific research in physics, nutrition, medicine, and psychology. You can trust that everything in our program is supported by science. What is new and exciting about our program comes out of the same basic research that brought you laser beams, microwaves, and nuclear energy.

A revolutionary concept, called *superstring theory,* has forced scientists to revise totally their understanding of the fundamental nature of matter and of life. This new theory has changed our ideas about the relationship between energy and health.

One of the problems with being "scientific" is that it's easy to view a human being as a machine that requires fuel, repair jobs, and supervision. All you have to do, according to this mechanistic view, is to figure out the right combination of things to do to the body. Then, like a machine, it will continue to function smoothly. Superstring theory has changed such ideas. It forces everyone in the field of preventive health care to see human beings in a totally new light, to recognize that each of us is a complex energy system capable of self-repair, of creating our own energy, and of controlling our own level of health and vitality.

The Never Be Tired Again program is the first to combine what we know about body chemistry with the incredible discoveries of quantum physics and the superstring hypothesis. As a result, this book will stretch your mind, challenge every idea you have about how your body works, and open your eyes to amazing secrets that will let you literally program yourself for health. And you don't need to understand physics in order to make this new knowledge work for you.

THE FOUR LEGS OF HIGH ENERGY

While we were doing our research into what makes some people tired all the time and what makes other people live long, healthy, energy-filled lives, we discovered that all our findings could be divided into four areas or methods. We call these the four legs of the energy chair. Just as a chair supports your weight, the four methods detailed in the following pages will support your health and energy levels. And just as with a chair, all four legs are equally important. We believe that each of the four methods will enhance your life. Together, they have incredible power to help in your transformation!

METHOD 1. HOW TO PROGRAM YOURSELF FOR HIGH ENERGY

We show you how to use three practical self-programming techniques to turn yourself into a human energy dynamo. These techniques are powerful because they help you harness the energy of quantum physics for your personal benefit. As you will see, all three are grounded in sophisticated physics research. However, the principles upon which the three programming techniques are based can be summarized in this simple phrase: *You are what you think.*

Because these easy-to-learn exercises are so effective, they form the essential core of the program. We call them "quick energy charges," and a quick energy charge is a vital component of almost every chapter in this book. They will help you get control of your life. They will also help you increase your performance, lower your blood pressure, and increase your ability to deal effectively with the stress in your life. These techniques are so relaxing and satisfying that after you have been using them for a while, you will wonder how you ever got along without them!

METHOD 2: THE NEVER BE TIRED AGAIN NUTRITION PROGRAM

We also tell you in lay language everything you need to know about high-energy nutrition:
- How to get more energy from food

- How to avoid foods that drain you of energy
- How to select foods that prevent disease

The Never Be Tired Again nutritional information and techniques are also based on research in high-energy physics. We believe that learning how to capitalize on what physics can teach you about your body as an energy-generating system is perhaps the most important part of our nutrition program. This section of the book contains simple and practical techniques to help you modify your diet without driving yourself up the wall.

METHOD 3: ENERGY-BUILDING EXERCISES

We will also help you develop your own exercise program, one that focuses on getting more oxygen into your system. Since oxygen is the key to energy production and storage, this program will help you increase your productivity and prevent tiredness. In addition, research has shown that these techniques help prevent heart disease and control stress and anxiety. The Never Be Tired Again exercise program is based on principles of high-energy physics that we like to summarize with the phrase *You are what you choose to do*.

The exercise program you set up for yourself will determine how well your body and mind function. The program's positive effects on your energy level are astounding. For most people, the effects are felt within days. Graduate after graduate of our program talks about being able to stick with the exercise program because of how energetic, creative, patient, and productive it makes one feel on days when one exercises, as opposed to days when one doesn't. We have included some new self-programming techniques that will help you over the hump that lies between being a "couch potato" and being a trim, energy-packed person.

METHOD 4: BREATH DYNAMICS

Most people are on autopilot most of the time. Think of your body as a modern jet plane: It can be flown by the pilot (your conscious mind) or by the autopilot mechanism (your autonomic nervous system). This is particularly true when it comes to your respiratory system. Here you truly have a choice. You can consciously control your breath or let it run on autopilot. But if your autopilot is improperly programmed, you may not be getting enough oxygen. Not getting enough oxygen sharply cuts the amount of energy your body can produce. The more oxygen you can breathe in efficiently, the more energy molecules you can manufacture and store.

With this in mind, we provide an overview of the art and science of breath control. The scientifically established benefits of respiratory training and control include getting more oxygenated blood into your energy system; helping to control your stress level; improving your bowel function; and, last but not least in these days of immune system diseases, *helping to strengthen your immune system*. We have also integrated breath control experiences into the Quick Energy Charges at the end of most chapters. The end result will be that you will learn how to reach incredible energy "highs" by consciously flying your own imaginary jet plane. In addition you will spontaneously improve the programming of your respiratory system's autopilot so it too will work more efficiently.

HOW TO GET STARTED ON THE SEVEN-DAY PROGRAM

This book is organized in such a way that you can begin our program without knowing all of the details about why it works. All you have to do is follow the seven-day program outlined in chapter 10, where you will find step-by-step directions for duplicating each step of our live-in program. Chapter 10 includes a schedule of activities, meals, and exercises for the entire period. Later on in the book we also provide recipes for each day. If you want to follow the seven-day start-up program completely, you may want to schedule a special week in your life to get started.

DOING IT YOUR WAY IS OKAY

It is not necessary for you to start off with our seven-day schedule to get results. If you want to start more gradually, by all means do so. There is no need to hurry, and each small step you take to change your lifestyle will increase your energy level. As you begin to feel more energetic and more in control, you can incorporate more of the program into your lifestyle. Take it easy, go step by step, each day substituting a new good habit or choice for an old, poor one.

Above all, *focus on increasing your level of awareness of your choices.* Live each moment as much as possible in the conscious thought that you can and will improve your energy and your health so that the promise of this book will come true for you—that you will never be tired again.

Chapter 2

Where Are You Now?
Assessing Your Lifestyle

Recently Harry, an acquaintance of ours, had a heart attack severe enough to put him in an intensive care unit. For several days he walked a tightrope between life and death. The good news is that Harry pulled through and was able to convalesce at home. The sad news is that he could have avoided the heart attack altogether if, in previous years, he had chosen a different lifestyle.

Harry's experience highlights a significant but little-known health statistic: *Seventy percent of all Americans who spend time in an intensive care unit need not have been there at all.* That may sound incredible, but it is true. Most medical problems that require intensive care stem from preventable diseases directly related to the lifestyle choices each of us makes every day.

Harry's case is not unusual. Statistics predict that 45 percent of all Americans—virtually one of every two persons you know—will suffer some form of heart disease. However, this is not the end of Harry's story. At the time he had his heart attack he was also being treated for cancer. Again, not all that surprising, since statistics show that 23 percent of all Americans will contract some form of that disease. Yet cancers, like heart disease and other potential killers such as hypertension, stroke, and adult-onset diabetes, are lifestyle-associated and to a great extent preventable.

Unfortunately, we aren't through with Harry's story yet. It is common knowledge today that good nutrition is a key factor in the prevention of lifestyle-associated ailments. Yet when Harry came out of intensive care, the first meal he was served consisted of steak, a baked potato with gravy, and a glass of milk. And Harry was being treated in a well-known, top-rated medical facility! It is hard to believe that this high-fat, high-protein meal was served to a man who had both cancer and heart disease, when research consistently shows that a high-fat, high-protein diet may be linked to the development of cancer and heart disease! Here is one more example of the current medical mind-set that all too often is willing to pour millions of dollars into the treatment of disease but scarcely any into prevention.

IS YOUR LIFESTYLE ENHANCING OR WEAKENING YOUR ENERGY LEVEL?

Do you feel that you face the same risks as Harry? Or does your way of living provide the high level of energy that enables you to lower those risks?

To help you discover how your lifestyle impacts your health and your energy level, we have developed a scientifically valid *High-Energy Lifestyle Inventory* (HELI).[1] This measures how effectively your present way of life provides you with the high energy flows that undergird good health. Its eighty items cover four basic lifestyle areas: your physical condition; your reactions to common situations at work, at home, or with friends; your psychological attitudes and emotional behavior; and your feelings about personal relationships. In addition, the HELI measures the degree of stress you feel you are under, and other medical-psychological factors that research shows may affect your general health and energy level.

Since the HELI is a self-report questionnaire, it can only be as accurate as the information you provide. However, we spent four years developing the inventory and tested it with thousands of people to ensure its accuracy and to make certain each item meets rigorous standards of validity.

The items on the survey were compiled during four years of research and pilot testing in our work with individuals and corporations. The final instrument has reliability and validity data that puts the HELI in a league with established psychological inventories.

In the latest round of research completed in 1987, the inventory was mailed to 30,000 people in key high-density popula-

---

[1] Gardner, D.C., and Beatty, G. J., "How Fit Are Americans?" Research paper presented at the annual convention of the American Board of Medical Psychotherapists, Cancun, Mexico, May 1987.

tion cities: New York, Boston, Dallas, Chicago, San Francisco, and Los Angeles. The 30,000 names were selected at random from an initial pool of 100,000, and 4,393 returns were received on the first mailing. This yielded a return rate of 14.6 percent. Subsequent follow-up studies of nonrespondents found the sample to be representative of the original population pool of 100,000. The research on the HELI was reviewed by a panel of experts from the American Board of Medical Psychotherapists and subsequently selected for presentation at their annual convention in 1987. As a result, the HELI can be considered a reasonably correct assessment of one's lifestyle.

A computer analysis of the returns indicated that roughly 50 percent of respondents fell into the high-risk category. Of this group, 55 percent were in the high-risk category for arthritis, 45 percent for heart ailments, 43 percent for high blood pressure, and 29 percent for cancer. (You will notice that the figures add up to more than 100 percent. This is because some people were in the high-risk category for several diseases.) These are frightening statistics. They clearly indicate a widespread need for lifestyle assessment and lifestyle change.

To find out if your lifestyle generates enough energy so that your body can protect itself against disease, complete every item in the following HELI. (*Note:* The HELI is not meant to take the place of a physical examination. If you have any concerns about your health we urge you to consult your physician.)

THE HIGH-ENERGY LIFESTYLE INVENTORY

I. Physical Aging

Directions: Listed below are some symptoms, situations, and behaviors you may experience. For convenience in using, photocopy this and the subsequent inventory items in this chapter. For each item, circle the number on the scale that best represents the extent to which you agree or disagree with each statement. Thus, if you agree completely with a statement, circle the number closest to that end of the scale; if you disagree completely, circle the number closest to the "disagree" end of the scale. If you agree or disagree partially, circle the number that most closely represents the strength of your feeling. If you feel neutral about a statement, circle number 4. Be sure to answer each item. Remember, there are no "right" or "wrong" answers; what matters is your opinion.

1. I get pains in my chest but my heart is fine. Disagree 7 6 5 4 3 2 1 Agree

2. I have trouble catching my breath. Disagree 7 6 5 4 3 2 1 Agree

3. I have headaches. Disagree 7 6 5 4 3 2 1 Agree

4. I have to urinate frequently. Disagree 7 6 5 4 3 2 1 Agree

5. I have no appetite (or I eat all the time). Disagree 7 6 5 4 3 2 1 Agree

6. I get dizzy for no reason. Disagree 7 6 5 4 3 2 1 Agree

7. I spend my nights awake, or it takes forever to fall asleep. Disagree 7 6 5 4 3 2 1 Agree

8. I'm tired. Disagree 7 6 5 4 3 2 1 Agree

9. My throat and/or mouth is often dry. Disagree 7 6 5 4 3 2 1 Agree

10. I sigh a lot. Disagree 7 6 5 4 3 2 1 Agree

11. My stomach is tense. Disagree 7 6 5 4 3 2 1 Agree

12. I have no energy. Disagree 7 6 5 4 3 2 1 Agree

13. I'm chilly. Disagree 7 6 5 4 3 2 1 Agree

14. I actually throw up for no reason. Disagree 7 6 5 4 3 2 1 Agree

15. My neck (or shoulders, eyes, chest, lower back, hands, throat) is sore, stiff, or painful Disagree 7 6 5 4 3 2 1 Agree

16. Lately I seem to have one bug or cold after another. Disagree 7 6 5 4 3 2 1 Agree

17. In the afternoon I run out of steam. Disagree 7 6 5 4 3 2 1 Agree

18. My posture is terrible. Disagree 7 6 5 4 3 2 1 Agree

19. I eat very little breakfast or lunch, and most of my calories are eaten in the evening. Disagree 7 6 5 4 3 2 1 Agree

20. I can bend over and touch my toes easily without hurting my back. Disagree 1 2 3 4 5 6 7 Agree

21. I can walk up a flight of stairs without puffing. Disagree 1 2 3 4 5 6 7 Agree

22. I don't have more than seven drinks a week, and not more than two at any one time. Disagree 1 2 3 4 5 6 7 Agree

23. I get at least seven hours sleep a night. Disagree 1 2 3 4 5 6 7 Agree

24. I eat very little red meat, fried food, or other fatty foods. Disagree 1 2 3 4 5 6 7 Agree

25. I eat lots of fresh fruits, vegetables, and whole grains every day. Disagree 1 2 3 4 5 6 7 Agree

26. I avoid white sugar, salt, and "junk food." Disagree 1 2 3 4 5 6 7 Agree

27. Most people think I am younger than I am. Disagree 1 2 3 4 5 6 7 Agree

28. I do some form of cardiovascular fitness exercise at least four times a week for at least twenty minutes each time.

Disagree 1 2 3 4 5 6 7 Agree

29. I have a lot of energy.

Disagree 1 2 3 4 5 6 7 Agree

30. I enjoy a day of vigorous physical activity.

Disagree 1 2 3 4 5 6 7 Agree

31. When necessary, I can work long hours without getting moody, overtired or cranky.

Disagree 1 2 3 4 5 6 7 Agree

Add up your ratings for items 1 to 31. Then match your score with its appropriate energy/risk level.

Score	Energy/Risk Level
31–139	Low energy, high risk
140–184	Average energy, medium risk
185–217	High energy, low risk

Your score indicates how well you are aging physically. This in turn affects your energy level and your physical health. The lower your score, the more we would be willing to bet that you look older than you are, that you feel older than you are, that most of the time you drag yourself through your day and that, to sum up, you're not having a whole lot of fun in life any more.

Low physical aging scores (31–139) are associated with:

High blood pressure	**Ulcers**
Heart disease	**Gout**
Inability to trust	**Feelings of unhappiness**
Smoking	**Being overweight**
Feeling overstressed	**Having a waist larger than your hips**

Average physical aging scores (140–184):
Don't be lulled into complacency by an "average" score. Remember that, *on the average, almost one out of two Americans has heart disease and one out of four has some form of cancer.* The best way to interpret a medium-risk score is to measure it against the high- and low-range scores. The closer your score is to the high-energy category, the more likely it is that you can join the ranks of the high scorers. Conversely, the lower your score, the more likely you are to end up with one or more of the health problems in the low-energy category if you don't change your lifestyle.

High physical aging scores (185–217) are associated with:

Good physical health	**Good mental health**
Healthy weight level	**Having a waist smaller than your**
Good relationships	**hips**
	Being in charge of your health

Individual Subscores to Focus on in This Scale

The total of all items in the physical aging scale is a good predictor of whether your lifestyle is an energy-producing one in a physical sense. But there are two subgroups of specific test items that should be interpreted individually even if your total score was in the high range:

NUTRITION SUBSCORE

Circle your ratings on items 22, 24, 25, and 26. Add them together and divide the total by 4. This is your nutrition subscore. This score should not be below 5. Next, examine each item separately. For optimum energy and health, no single rating should be below 5. Write down your nutrition subscore.

PHYSICAL ACTIVITY SUBSCORE

Note your ratings on items 20, 21, 28, and 30. Add them together and divide the total by 4. This is your physical activity subscore. This score should not be below 5. Next, examine each item separately. No single rating should be below 5 for optimum energy and health. To help prevent heart disease, you should strive to have item 28 rated a 7. As you will see in chapter 18, cardiovascular exercise four times a week is essential to maintaining a high-energy lifestyle. Write down your physical activity subscore.

II. Your Behaviors

DIRECTIONS: Listed below are some common situations that may occur at work, at home, or socially. Think for a minute about how you have behaved in the past in similar situations. Then indicate on your photocopy how you think you have behaved or would behave in the future.

32. The next outfit I buy will be the one I like best, regardless of what fashion designers are offering.   Disagree 1 2 3 4 5 6 7 Agree

33. The next time I'm involved in a disagreement, I will make every effort to get the issues out on the table rather than letting things clear up on their own.

Disagree 1 2 3 4 5 6 7 Agree

34. When I work on a difficult project, I try to do it myself rather than ask for help.

Disagree 1 2 3 4 5 6 7 Agree

35. The last time I finished a project successfully I couldn't wait for my coworkers to tell me how good it was.

Disagree 7 6 5 4 3 2 1 Agree

36. I prefer TV shows in which the hero works on his own.

Disagree 1 2 3 4 5 6 7 Agree

37. When I misunderstand people, it's usually their fault because they don't explain themselves enough.

Disagree 7 6 5 4 3 2 1 Agree

38. I always do my best work regardless of other people's performance.

Disagree 1 2 3 4 5 6 7 Agree

39. The last time I got a raise, I said to myself, "Boy, it's about time; I sure earned this one."

Disagree 1 2 3 4 5 6 7 Agree

40. I have always believed that my career success is directly related to my own efforts.

Disagree 1 2 3 4 5 6 7 Agree

41. If I hear that someone has made negative comments about me, I worry that other people may be thinking the same thing.

Disagree 7 6 5 4 3 2 1 Agree

Add up your ratings for items 32 to 41. Then match your score with its appropriate energy/risk level.

Score	Energy/Risk Level
10–40	Low energy, high risk
41–62	Average energy, medium risk
63–70	High energy, low risk

What do you think is the most common characteristic of people who stay healthy or who live well into old age? It is a strong belief in personal control. There is no doubt that healthy, long-lived people are in charge of their lives until the day they die! Consequently, they score in the very high range on the Behavior Scale and other tests like it.

In terms of your own life, the more you operate from a belief in personal control, the more successful, healthy, and happy you will be. Over fifty years of social science research consistently proves that *people who believe that what happens to them is a result of their own actions do better at everything!* In contrast, if you blame all of your successes or failures on other, more powerful people or on luck, fate, or chance, we guarantee you will not be as healthy or happy as you could otherwise be. Amazingly, a belief in personal control makes a difference even with hospitalized patients. Studies show that patients who get actively involved in their own healing process are more likely to be cured. And what's more, they get well faster!

If you scored high on personal control, you are more likely to be physically fit. You probably have people in your life you can trust. And even if you are in a high-stress job or situation, you probably feel you can readily deal with that stress.

If you scored low on personal control, you need to examine your beliefs about personal responsibility. Do you believe that *you* are primarily responsible for the things—good or bad—that happen in your life? Or do you tend to believe that most things that happen to you are due to luck, fate, or because other people manipulated you into or out of something. Frankly, if you want to make real changes in your life, you need to start believing in your ability to control your own future. Those who don't often have trouble trusting people and tend to feel they are being used by others. They feel that stress is beyond their control.

Moreover, people who score low on belief in personal control report a higher incidence of family members with high blood pressure, heart disease, and cancer. While there is evidence that genetics is a factor in susceptibility to these diseases, we think it may be less of a factor than it seems at first glance. Suppose we look at the risk from the point of view of belief in personal control. Isn't it likely that high-risk people blame their genetic background for their physical condition? That they have a deep-seated belief that modern medicine (the powerful "others" in health care) can bail them out with a pill or an operation? Or perhaps they believe that whatever happens is predetermined by fate or the stars.

If you believe the key areas of your life are beyond your control, you are ignoring the fact that *you can make yourself healthier, have more energy, be more productive, and enjoy life more simply by taking personal responsibility for what happens to you.* By choosing to participate in your own life processes you can change yourself and your body.

Low behavior scores (10–40) are associated with:
Low levels of wellness
Not being physically fit
Inability to trust other people
Stress that seems out of control
High incidence of family members with high blood
     pressure, heart disease, and cancer

Average behavior scores (41–62):
The lower your score in this range, the more likely you are to end up with one or more of the health problems listed in the low-energy category. The name of the healthy, high-energy game is to take command of your life now!

High behavior scores (63–70) are associated with:
Healthy personal relationships
Ability to control stress in a healthy way
High levels of physical fitness
Normal weight
A high total high-energy lifestyle score (at the end of this
     inventory)

III.   Your Attitudes

DIRECTIONS: Listed below are some behaviors and/or attitudes that may apply to your everyday living. Please indicate on the scale for each item the degree to which you agree or disagree with the statement.

42. I have trouble concentrating on my work.   Disagree 7 6 5 4 3 2 1 Agree

43. I don't trust anybody.   Disagree 7 6 5 4 3 2 1 Agree

44. It takes me forever to make decisions   Disagree 7 6 5 4 3 2 1 Agree

45. From the time I get to work until I leave, I'm
     plain fidgety.   Disagree 7 6 5 4 3 2 1 Agree

46. I overreact to things at work.   Disagree 7 6 5 4 3 2 1 Agree

47. I let minor things get to me.   Disagree 7 6 5 4 3 2 1 Agree

48. I procrastinate.   Disagree 7 6 5 4 3 2 1 Agree

49. I can't seem to get organized.   Disagree 7 6 5 4 3 2 1 Agree

50. I don't seem to judge people right.   Disagree 7 6 5 4 3 2 1 Agree

51. I work long hours and bring work home.   Disagree 7 6 5 4 3 2 1 Agree

52. I do a lot of paper shuffling.   Disagree 7 6 5 4 3 2 1 Agree

53. I don't trust anyone at work.   Disagree 7 6 5 4 3 2 1 Agree

54. I work longer and harder than most other people.   Disagree 7 6 5 4 3 2 1 Agree

55. I'm very competitive at everything.   Disagree 7 6 5 4 3 2 1 Agree

Add up your ratings for items 42 to 55. Then match your score with its appropriate energy/risk level.

Score	Energy/Risk Level
14–59	Low energy, high risk
60–87	Average energy, medium risk
88–98	High energy, low risk

Do you know someone who sticks with a task or a job even if she hates it? Is that person often constipated? How about someone who always complains about how his parents neglected him or damaged his life? Does he have asthma? Do you know someone who believes he never gets what he deserves but somehow or other intends to get even? Does he have an ulcer? Do you know someone who constantly says she is "chained" to her job or marriage and can't do anything about it? Does she have rheumatoid arthritis?

What do all these people have in common? Simple. They are filtering their lives through a set of "attitudes" that research shows are associated with illness. Obviously, if you hold negative attitudes about yourself and your life, your subconscious is working against any positive changes you may want to implement.

Your score on the attitudes scale is a barometer of how your way of looking at things affects your energy and health. Although this area is controversial, the trend in current medical and psychological research supports the idea that certain positive attitudes are indeed associated with wellness. This makes a lot of sense. If you are generating negative thought-energy waves about yourself, you are bound to impact your body's energy system in an unhealthy way. Our research on a representative group of 4,393 Americans found that people who have difficulty trusting others are prone to have high blood pressure, heart disease, and ulcers. Their overall lifestyle works against their health.

We found that if your attitude score is high you tend to be trusting and to have a healthy outlook on competition. In other words, you can be competitive when you need to be, or you can work cooperatively when cooperation is appropriate. Being overly competitive can be counterproductive. An overly competitive, nontrusting set of attitudes produces a hard-driving person who doesn't know how to relax and so works to the point of exhaustion. This is classic Type A behavior, and heart attacks come with the territory! Fortunately, this kind of behavior can be modified if you make the effort. If you scored low on the attitude scale, you need to examine your life in the context of developing the ability to work cooperatively and to trust others.

Low attitude scores (14–59) are associated with:
   High blood pressure
   Heart disease
   Inability to relax
   Ulcers
   Arthritis
   Pushing too hard
   Counterproductive competitiveness
   Overall lifestyle that is energy-depleting
   Not being physically fit

Average attitude scores (60–87):
The best way to interpret an average attitude score is to compare it with the scores in the low and high ranges. The closer your score is to the high-energy category, the better your chances are of developing a set of attitudes that do not send negative, disease-generating thoughts into your energy system. You can enhance the process of developing more positive attitudes if you try harder to work cooperatively with those around you. You should make every effort to be involved with people in a mutually sharing and supportive environment.

The lower your average score, the higher the probability that you may end up with one or more of the health problems listed in the low-energy category. For example, if your answers indicate that you are overly competitive or have trouble trusting people, you run the risk of high blood pressure or heart disease. (We don't mean you will get a specific disease because you hold a specific attitude. What we mean is that *your risk* of getting these diseases is higher than it is for people who do not have these attitudes.) You need to practice letting go, to spend more time relaxing. Remember, you have the power to change all the probabilities of your future by the choices that you make now!

High attitude scores (88–98) are associated with:
   A healthy attitude towards competitiveness
   Ability to work in a more cooperative mode when appropriate
   Being physically fit
   Overall, a health- and energy-producing lifestyle

IV. Your Relationships

DIRECTIONS: Listed below are some feelings and attitudes that you may hold at times about yourself or others. Please indicate on the scale for each item the degree to which you agree or disagree with the statement.

56. I startle easily when people come up on me.   Disagree 7 6 5 4 3 2 1 Agree

57. I can't stand to be around a particular person (or group)   Disagree 7 6 5 4 3 2 1 Agree

58. I can't stand to be around people when they are emotional.   Disagree 7 6 5 4 3 2 1 Agree

59. I can't tell anyone how I feel.   Disagree 7 6 5 4 3 2 1 Agree

60. I don't feel anything.   Disagree 7 6 5 4 3 2 1 Agree

61. I worry a lot.   Disagree 7 6 5 4 3 2 1 Agree

62. I feel unhappy.   Disagree 7 6 5 4 3 2 1 Agree

63. I imagine scary things.   Disagree 7 6 5 4 3 2 1 Agree

64. There are times when I can't react to anything; I'm frozen in time and space.   Disagree 7 6 5 4 3 2 1 Agree

65. Life seems so unreal.   Disagree 7 6 5 4 3 2 1 Agree

66. I don't know what's the matter with me. I'm so irritable all the time.   Disagree 7 6 5 4 3 2 1 Agree

67. I feel like I'm living inside a pressure cooker and am about to explode.   Disagree 7 6 5 4 3 2 1 Agree

68. I've finally realized that people use me all the time.   Disagree 7 6 5 4 3 2 1 Agree

69. Lately I'm bored with my life, my job, my friends, and even my loved ones.

Disagree 7 6 5 4 3 2 1 Agree

70. Deep inside, I'm dissatisfied and I don't know why.

Disagree 7 6 5 4 3 2 1 Agree

71 I forget things.

Disagree 7 6 5 4 3 2 1 Agree

72. When I get up in the morning, I look forward to the day ahead.

Disagree 1 2 3 4 5 6 7 Agree

73. I feel in control of my life most of the time.

Disagree 1 2 3 4 5 6 7 Agree

74. I have good friends and an active social life.

Disagree 1 2 3 4 5 6 7 Agree

75. I am good at what I do.

Disagree 1 2 3 4 5 6 7 Agree

76. I enjoy learning and doing new things.

Disagree 1 2 3 4 5 6 7 Agree

77. I have a new career, hobby, or personal goal for next year.

Disagree 1 2 3 4 5 6 7 Agree

78. There are times when I feel like crying for no reason.

Disagree 7 6 5 4 3 2 1 Agree

79. I like to have people of all ages involved in my life.

Disagree 1 2 3 4 5 6 7 Agree

80. I enjoy physical activities.

Disagree 1 2 3 4 5 6 7 Agree

Add up your ratings for items 56 to 80. Then match your score with its appropriate energy/risk level category.

Score	Energy/Risk Level
25–80	Low energy, high risk
81–159	Average energy, medium risk
160–175	High energy, low risk

In general, the higher you score on this scale the happier you are with your life and the more likely you are to have an energy-producing lifestyle. A high score also indicates that you handle the stress in your life well. *How you deal with stress is more important than the kind or amount of stress you are under.* People who have stress-related ailments do not necessarily have more stress in their lives than others; the difference is that they feel less in control of it and do not do a good job of managing the effect stress has on their bodies and minds.

We found that people who scored low on this scale reported significantly more family history of high blood pressure, heart disease, and cancer of the lung, colon, and reproductive organs than people who scored high. This puts low scorers at significantly greater risk because of the cumulative effect of a counterproductive lifestyle combined with this family medical background.

Low relationship scores (25–80) are associated with:
Ulcers
Heart disease
Colitis
Not being physically fit
Being unhappy with your life
Having an overall lifestyle that is energy-depleting
Smoking
A family history of heart disease, colon cancer, lung cancer, reproductive organ cancer

Average relationship scores (81–159):
Besides belief in personal control, can you think of another important characteristic of long-lived people? In our research we found that almost without exception long-lived people have highly supportive family and personal relationships. In fact, they have a wide social network. Keep this in mind when you interpret your "average relationship score." Ask yourself if you really want to be average.

The closer your score is to the high-energy category, the more likely you are to be able to develop some truly rewarding relationships if you are willing to work at expanding your social life and take more time to enjoy life. The lower your score, the greater the probability that you may develop one or more of the health problems listed in the low-energy category unless you begin to handle stress better. You probably need a vacation, just for starters!

High relationship scores (160–175) are associated with:
Being happy with your life in general
Having an overall lifestyle that is conducive to wellness
Being physically fit

V. Your Total High-Energy Lifestyle Score

To determine your total HELI score, write down your subscale scores and add them up.

Physical aging score
Behaviors score
Attitude score
Relationship score
Total high-energy lifestyle score

To determine your energy/risk level, compare your score with the following categories:

Score	Energy/Risk Level
80–325	Low energy, high risk
326–494	Average energy, medium risk
495–560	High energy, low risk

Low total scores (80–325) are associated with:
Ulcers
Heart Disease
Colitis
Cancer
Arthritis
Unhappiness
Inability to trust others
Energy-depleting stress that is out of control
Not accepting responsibility for your life
Not accepting responsibility for your health

Average total scores (326–494):
This category represents those in the middle. The best way to interpret an average total lifestyle score is to compare your actual score with the ranges for the high and low categories. The closer your score is to the high-energy category, the more likely you are to join the ranks of the high scorers—if you're willing to reexamine your total lifestyle and make energy-producing modifications. The lower your score, the higher the probability that, unless you take positive lifestyle steps, you risk developing one or more health problems that stem from a low-energy lifestyle. You can begin the process of consciously taking part in your lifestream process now! The techniques for doing this are detailed in the chapters that follow.

High total scores (495–560) are associated with:
Excellent physical condition
High levels of energy
High levels of health
Feelings of being in control of your life
Feelings of being in control of your health
Feeling satisfied with your life
Having excellent personal relationships and support system

IDENTIFYING AND CHANGING YOUR NEGATIVE ATTITUDES

Your individual scores on the various scales of the High-Energy Lifestyle Inventory, plus your total score, have given you a global look at where your lifestyle is leading you, for better or worse. What the scores don't do is pinpoint specific areas that need improvement. Fortunately, there is another way to use the HELI that will give you additional key insights. We think you will find the process easy and helpful.

Many of the items in the scales measure attitudes, or the way you feel and think about people and situations in your life. *Most of these attitudes are unconscious.* What this means is that you may be unwittingly creating—via self-defeating statements, beliefs, and attitudes—a reality that is not in your best interest. You may be your own worst enemy!

For example, item 75 asks you to rate the statement "I am good at what I do." If you rated yourself low on that item, it's almost certain that you will never be good at what you do! But you can change that reality by devising a plan of action that literally can create a new reality for yourself—one in which you truly *are* good at what you do. Such an action plan would be based on a combination of the techniques we discuss in Part III. For instance, you might begin a series of daily visualization exercises wherein you see yourself selected as "employee of the month." This technique can then be combined with a mindfulness or awareness activity at work, whereby you consciously observe yourself improving by quantum leaps while you perform your job.

HOW FAMILY BACKGROUND, ENVIRONMENT, AND LIFESTYLE INTERPLAY

There are other important factors not measured by the HELI. Over the past twenty years extensive research indicates how genetic factors, physical characteristics, and lifestyle, separately and in combination, may be predictive of major health problems. Below are some facts you may want to consider in evaluating your lifestyle status beyond the HELI scores. Note that when genetics is removed from the list, the vast majority of the remaining factors are directly under your control. It is our belief that you can avoid most of these ailments even if they are present in your family's medical history. In fact, we believe that many of the so-called genetic factors are not genetic at all, but a result of an unhealthy, energy-depleting lifestyle that a family unwittingly passes on to the next generation. Remember, what grandma taught you ain't necessarily so!

SMOKING AND HEALTH

The link between smoking and health problems is well documented. Smokers are sick more often than nonsmokers. They are more likely to be unhappy with their lives, to have more difficulty trusting others, to experience more severe stress levels, and to be less accepting of responsibility for their health. It is not surprising that in our surveys smokers also had the lowest Total High-Energy Lifestyle and physical fitness scores. Research shows that about one out of two smokers will die as a direct result of smoking.

WEIGHT AND HEALTH

Research shows that overweight people are prone to heart disease, cancer, and adult-onset diabetes, among other diseases. Overweight men are more than twice as likely to get prostate cancer than men who are not overweight.

WAIST AND HIP MEASUREMENTS

Measure your waist. Then measure your hips. Which is larger? A growing body of research indicates that if your waist is larger than your hips (even if you are not overweight), you have a greater chance of heart problems, stroke, hypertension, diabetes, gallbladder disease, and menstrual disorders.

CANCER

Twenty-three percent of all Americans can expect to get cancer. The most prevalent kinds of cancer for men are those of the lung and prostate, followed by cancer of the colon and bladder. For women the most prevalent forms are breast and lung cancer, followed by cancer of the uterus and colon. In our study, cancer was found to be associated with being too competitive, working too hard, finding it difficult to trust people, and not being physically fit. Cancer was also associated with a low Total High-Energy Lifestyle score—being overweight, having a waist larger than the hips, smoking, not accepting responsibility for one's own health, and having a family history of cancer. For instance, women whose mothers or sisters have or had breast cancer run more than twice the risk of getting the disease themselves. Having close relatives with colon cancer increases the risk four-fold. Men with close relatives who have or had prostate cancer run three to six times the risk of getting the disease than other men. Overweight men who eat meat, milk, cheese, and eggs more than triple their risk of prostate cancer.

Significantly, the incidence of cancer increases as one's socioeconomic status rises. Our clinical experience suggests that this is related to the fact that well-to-do men and women tend to eat a diet higher in fats. In fact, it was not unusual to find, through a computerized nutritional analysis of clients in our live-in program, that many of our more affluent clients ate a diet close to 70 percent fat.

HEART DISEASE/STROKE

In our research, people with heart disease tended to smoke, have a family history of the ailment, be overweight, have a waist larger than the hips, have a low Total High-Energy Lifestyle score, and have an unhealthy level of stress. In our national study we found heart disease was also related to being unable to trust people, to feelings of unhappiness, and to not accepting responsibility for one's health.

HIGH BLOOD PRESSURE

We also found, in our research, that high blood pressure was related to the inability to trust, being overweight, poor physical condition, having a waist larger than the hips, a family history of high blood pressure, and being unhappy with one's life.

ARTHRITIS

Our study of 4,393 people showed arthritis correlates with being overweight, high stress, a low physical fitness level, smoking, living and working in an urban area, and not accepting responsibility for one's health.

DIABETES

Diabetes appears to be associated with stress, being overweight, a large waist, high competitiveness, a low level of trust, and with high blood pressure. Other research shows that diabetic men run a 70 percent greater risk of coronary heart disease, and diabetic women run a 200 percent greater risk. Yet in many cases adult-onset diabetes can be arrested and controlled by lifestyle changes.

ULCERS

Not surprisingly, ulcers are directly related to stress, to working in an urban area, to being overweight, and to not accepting responsibility for one's health.

YOU CAN MODIFY YOUR GENETIC RISK FACTORS

If you are like most people, somewhere amid the "gloom and doom" of the HELI testing or the discussion of genetic-environmental factors in disease, you probably found that you had at least one or more risk factors for a major lifestyle ailment. We share that scenario with you. David's genetic risk factor on both sides of his family includes the early death of male relatives from heart attacks, diabetes and cancer. Joely's risk factors include living in an urban area (until we made a change five years ago), a family history of cancer and arthritis, and heart disease among women on one side of her family.

Does this mean that David is going to drop dead of a heart attack like his father, uncles, and grandfather? Does this mean that Joely is going to get arthritis?

Absolutely not!

The difference is that both of us live our high-energy program lifestyle. It's easy and it works. You can do it, too! Before you read more of this book, take a moment and draft a list of things you think you need to change in your life in order to have more energy and never to be tired again. We show you how below.

DRAFTING YOUR PROPOSED LIFESTYLE CHANGE LIST

Take the time to think about the ratings you gave the statements in each section of the High-Energy Lifestyle Inventory. Then make a list of everything you think needs to be modified or changed as part of your Never Be Tired Again program. Make a list of any new behaviors you think you need to develop. For example, if your nutrition subscore is 5 or lower, you undoubtedly will have to get rid of some old eating habits and acquire newer, healthier ones. At this point your list need not be comprehensive. For now, think of it as a draft, a list that will grow and take shape as you learn more from the following chapters.

Chapter 3

Why Most People Are Tired All the Time

"Boy, am I beat! It's been a really rough day."

"Can't we stay home tonight, darling? I'm exhausted!"

"I don't understand it—I had seven solid hours of sleep and I wake up feeling exhausted."

"Nothing's really wrong with me, doctor . . . it's just that I don't seem to have much energy any more."

How often have you heard people say things like that? How often have you said them—or words much like them—yourself? Probably quite often, or you would not have picked up this book, hoping to learn how to get rid of that draining and depressing burden of fatigue.

If you are like most people, gathering the energy to do all the enjoyable things you *want* to do is often a wistful dream.

Copy the chart that follows in your Never Be Tired Again notebook, and complete the following "How Tired Am I?" checklist to get a picture of your energy level. There isn't any "official" score or rating, so you can be completely honest with yourself.

The purpose of the checklist is two-fold. First, to bring home to you sharply how much of your life is spent in a deenergized, unfulfilled physical and mental state. Second, to point out to you that "tiredness" is a highly individualized, personal condition. Being tired is a feeling that defies scientific description, definition, comparison, or measurement. The words *you* use to describe your feeling of tiredness can in no way match the actual feeling or be compared to some other person's feeling of tiredness.

THE "HOW TIRED AM I?" CHECKLIST

Simply put a check next to the words that best describe how you feel, in the column that best describes how often you feel that way.

	Some of the time	A lot of the time	Most of the time
pooped			
sleepy			
burnt out			
drawn			
fatigued			
run down			
worn out			
dull			
haggard			
listless			
lethargic			
beat			
bushed			
exhausted			
shot			
weary			
worn down			
stale			
frazzled			
sluggish			

A DEFINITION OF CHRONIC TIREDNESS

Chronic tiredness is a complex, frustrating, multifaceted problem that does not always lend itself to standard medical or psychological procedures and treatment. Chronic tiredness is a feeling you have with you most of the time. It is a feeling that you simply do not have enough energy to do the ordinary chores and tasks of your life. It includes a strong desire to stop all activity and just rest. People who suffer from severe chronic tiredness have difficulty with complex tasks. They may also experience personality changes such as becoming more unreasonable and short tempered as they feel more tired.

You will note that this definition *excludes* the kind of normal tiredness that comes from lack of sleep and/or heavy physical exertion. That is natural and usually can be remedied with a good night's sleep. Our definition also excludes tiredness that results from medical illness. If your chronic tiredness is not the result of medical problems, this is your opportunity to use our proven methods to manage your life so that you get more energy from every possible source each and every day. It is your opportunity to feel the sheer joy of being alive again.

THE PHYSICAL CAUSES OF TIREDNESS

YOUR FAVORITE FOODS CAN BE WEARING YOU OUT!

You get energy from the food you eat, but many people do not realize that some foods actually can sap your energy. This occurs when you are sensitive to a particular food or foods.

"But I'm not allergic to any food, so that can't be my problem," you say. Wrong! There is a big difference between *food allergy* and *food sensitivity*. An allergic reaction to food immediately triggers an immune system response—you cough, sneeze, break out in rashes or hives, have internal digestive disturbances, and more. There is a recognizable cause and effect relationship every time between the offending food and your usually rapid physical reaction.

Food sensitivities are a different matter altogether. They were originally labeled "masked allergies" because the reaction to the offending food does not occur immediately. Indeed, a person who is sensitive to a certain food may even feel better just after eating that food! This may seem contradictory, but examined in the light of the biochemistry of your body's stress response it makes sense. The first feeling you get when the stress response is triggered is one of being energized! The hormones pouring into your bloodstream are designed to get you ready for "fight or flight." In the case of a food sensitivity reaction, it is only later—when the body is overburdened in trying to deal with the offending food—that the negative symptoms show up. *This reaction can occur as late as three to five days after eating the food.* Typical symptoms of a food sensitivity reaction are:

- Chronic tiredness that doesn't go away after a good night's sleep
- Headaches, chest pains
- Mucus secretion, sneezing, runny nose
- Embarrassing conditions: abdominal gas pains, excessive flatulence, diarrhea
- Embarrassing eruptions: rash, skin irritations, eczema

The important point is that masked food sensitivities take time and effort to identify and correct. One method is to exclude the suspected food from your diet for five days. If your symptoms disappear, add the food back in and see what happens. This complicated routine must be repeated for each food. Another method is to fast (this requires medical supervision) for five days until all symptoms disappear. If you feel highly energetic during this time, chances are that all your symptoms may be related to food sensitivities. As in the previous method, you then add the suspected foods back into your diet one at a time and watch your body's reaction. Again, this is a time-consuming method.

A third technique for identifying food sensitivities is called the cytotoxic blood test. It was developed by a husband and wife team of doctors at Washington University School of Medicine in St. Louis. Some practitioners swear by it; others claim the test is not accurate. Research supports both sides, with most of the studies being favorable. Obviously, a simple blood test—if accurate—is preferable to fasting as a diagnostic method. We tried it ourselves, and it worked for us: It confirmed the food sensitivities that we had already verified via the fasting method. (To learn more about this method, we suggest you read *The Food Sensitivity Diet*, a book by Doug A. Kaufmann, PaperJacks, Ltd., 1986.)

If you think you may be sensitive to certain foods, make a list of the foods you eat most often—the ones you crave. Chances are they will be the offenders. The most common "masked foods" are wheat, corn, tomatoes, cane sugar, chocolate, fish, chicken, cow's milk, yeast, cheese, bacon, artificial food additives, and colorings.

MOM'S COOKING CAN SAP YOUR ENERGY

Our parents made a special effort to provide us with good nutrition. It wasn't their fault that the nutritional knowledge of the day defined healthy meals as those that included meat, potatoes, cream, cheese, butter, and white bread. Even today, some print advertisements and television commercials claim that sugar is an excellent source of quick energy, and that candy bars are good for a quick energy boost. Modern nutritional research has found that a diet like this is wrong. A diet high in fat, sugar, and protein and low in complex carbohydrates and fiber not only robs your body of essential vitamins and minerals but can accelerate a tendency to serious diseases—cancer, high blood pressure, heart problems, clogged arteries, diabetes, osteoporosis, and arthritis. Moreover, such a diet leaves you feeling sluggish. Your body has to work so hard to get the toxins of a high-protein, high-fat diet out of your system that there is little energy left for you to use to get through your everyday tasks. Part II of this book contains all the information you need to know to develop your own high-energy nutritional program.

WOMEN, NUTRITION, AND ENERGY

A pregnant or nursing mother is usually put on a special nutritional program. But does a nonpregnant woman who is not nursing have different nutritional needs from those of a man in terms of energy production? Fundamentally, no. The Never Be Tired Again nutritional program outlined in Part II works well for both sexes in terms of energy.

YOUR THIRST QUENCHERS MAY BE MAKING YOU TIRED

Most soft drinks are loaded with sugar, which puts a severe strain on the immune system and ultimately contributes to chronic tiredness. "But I use only sugar-free soft drinks," you say. Unfortunately, that doesn't get you off the hook. *Artificial colorings, flavorings, and sweeteners abound in soft drinks, and all of these substances drain energy.*

What about coffee? Because the caffeine in coffee overstimulates the immune system, you feel energetic soon after drinking it. But the effect is short-lived; you quickly crash. So you pour yourself another cup. And soon another. Eventually your system gets worn down by the constant stimulation of your fight-or-flight response. This yo-yo process not only leaves you tired and sluggish, it also weakens your immune system. If you have the self-discipline to be moderate in your coffee drinking, you can follow the advice of Judith Wurtman, Ph.D., in her book, *Managing Your*

Mind and Mood Through Food (Rawson Associates, 1986). According to the research done by Dr. Wurtman and her colleagues at the Massachusetts Institute of Technology, one to two cups of coffee or tea in the morning and one cup at 3:30 to 4:30 in the afternoon will improve your mental functioning and help you stay alert. Additional coffee will *not* give you increased benefits and definitely increases your risk of suffering from the potential side effects of caffeine consumption that we mentioned above. You can get the same benefits of alertness and increased mental functioning from the techniques outlined in the Never Be Tired Again program, without the potential risk associated with caffeine. So our recommendation is negative for the caffeine in coffee, tea, chocolate, and soft drinks.

CENTRAL HEATING AND AIRPLANES CAN MAKE YOU EXHAUSTED

Much of our tired feeling, experts say, comes from the loss of body fluids as we go through our daily routine. You can lose body fluids simply from being in the dry-air atmosphere of your office or home, or from flying in an airplane. Drinking caffeinated beverages or alcohol will not replenish or prevent the loss of these fluids. In fact, drinking these beverages contributes to the dehydration process because they act as diuretics. You can prevent the tiredness that comes from the loss of body fluids by drinking eight to twelve glasses of pure water a day. We suggest drinking carbonated pure spring water rather than tap water. Carbonated water is absorbed into your system faster; the gas bubbles help speed up the absorption process. We suggest you drink the low-sodium, naturally carbonated waters that are widely available now.

SITTING AND RIDING MAKE YOU SLUGGISH

Unless you have spent the last ten years in solitary confinement, you know that you should be exercising for heart health and weight control. Sitting around in your office or your car, even if you are not working hard mentally, makes you tired. The muscle tension generated by seated postures, especially under stressful conditions, can result in the physical exhaustion of your muscles. Whether you are working at a desk or at the kitchen table makes no difference. Even though you are performing a sedentary task you are actually stimulating and using the muscles in your upper back, neck, shoulders, face, and forehead—and probably tensing them more than usual. This tension squeezes the muscle and reduces the amount of blood and oxygen that can flow through the muscle. The decrease in blood and oxygen means that there is less nourishment for the muscle and less opportunity for waste products such as lactic acid to be carried out of the muscles. The Never Be Tired Again exercise program in Part IV is designed to help increase the amount of oxygen and blood that gets to your muscles and to create an abundance of energy.

WOMEN AND EXERCISE

Does the tired housewife syndrome mean that women have special problems? The answer is no. When Evalyn S. Gendel, M.D., studied the physical fitness of a group of one hundred women, she found that the more physically active women (not athletes, mind you) complained less about tiredness, allergies, digestive problems, and other ailments. Women (like men) who are physically active have more energy and fewer health problems. Not surprising. The real difference between men and women, Dr. Gendel believes, is how they are treated by the medical establishment. If a man complains to his doctor of chronic tiredness, according to Dr. Gendel, he "gets cured (put on a physical fitness program), and the woman gets tranquilized."

THE BRAIN DRAIN

Your brain needs a lot of high-octane fuel in the form of oxygen for peak performance. When your blood supply is low on oxygen, your brain starts to "ping" like a poorly tuned car engine. It loses its power, and you are not as sharp and productive as you might be. The key to preventing a tired brain is learning how to get more oxygen from exercise, from food, and—this may surprise you—from learning how to breathe more efficiently. (We'll show you how to do this later in this book.) Increased oxygen utilization is a primary focus of the Never Be Tired program.

YOUR BODY RHYTHMS AND CYCLES

You probably pay little attention to natural and bodily rhythms until you take a long-distance airplane flight. Suddenly your biological systems are out of sync, out of rhythm, totally confused. You're sleepy when you should be wide awake and wide awake when you should be asleep; your digestive and elimination systems are upset; your thinking and productivity are slowed down. If you stay in your new location long enough, your inner time clock will readjust itself to the new cycle. But it can take as long as three weeks before you return to your normal energy level.

Rhythms or cycles are found in all living things. For humans, the most basic one is called the circadian, or twenty-four-hour, cycle. Tied to the daily rotation of the earth (day/night, sleep/wake cycle), it has a profound impact on our lives. In terms of tiredness and energy, this endless cycle guarantees that at some point in the twenty-four hours you will be more tired than at other times. Your mood will change, and your blood pressure will vary according to the cycle. Your body temperature, your hormone levels, your performance, and your pulse are all affected by this daily cycle. Your energy level will rise and fall during each rotation of the earth.

Within the circadian cycle there are individual differences. Some of us are early birds, and some of us are night owls. Since our nine-to-five world does not take this into account, many of us must work when we feel sluggish and tired, and then try to go to sleep when we feel energized.

Other familiar cycles also affect us. It does not require a scientific survey to point out the difference in mood, energy level, and appetite that a woman may often exhibit before, during, and after her monthly period, or to note that this cycle can have a profound affect on her behavior. (Incidentally, there is some evidence that men go through a similar monthly cycle.)

In addition to daily and monthly rhythms, humans are also affected by the cycles of the four seasons. Take, for example, the onset of spring fever. With the advent of spring your body prepares to lower its temperature in response to the warmer spring air. In essence, your blood is thinning. *While this biochemical process is going on, you experience a temporary energy deficit.* Conversely, did you ever notice how much more energy you have in summer if the temperature isn't too hot? That's because you are getting more natural light than during the winter. Natural light increases energy and performance. After reading the research on this scientific finding, we put full-spectrum lighting in our office because it is the next best thing to natural light. It makes a huge difference in our energy and performance levels. Some people are so negatively affected by the seasonal decline of natural (sun) light that they experience severe depression during fall and winter and "highs" during the spring and summer. This phenomenon is called seasonal affective disorder (SAD). The preferred treatment is phototherapy (light therapy).

Surgeons have long known that the flow of blood in the human body is affected by the phases of the moon. Some surgeons will not operate during a full moon because they know they are going to get bleeders. This makes sense when you realize that your body is 80 percent water, just as affected by lunar cycles as the tides in the ocean! A few researchers have compiled evidence that leads them to believe that aggressive behavior and violent crime are also linked to the full moon and lunar rhythms. Studies show definite correlations between solar activities such as sunspots and human blood cell counts, the incidence of epidemics, sudden death rates, and nervous breakdowns.

Try to be more aware of the times of day when you experience energy peaks and valleys. Eating one of the recommended snacks in the seven-day program will help you over a low spot. Following the specific suggestions in this book for high-energy exercises and nutrition will help you eliminate the valleys and accentuate the peaks.

SPEAKING OF YOUR ENVIRONMENT

We recommend "living in the light" as much as possible. If you do not live in an area that gets a lot of sunshine, by all means equip your office and home with full-spectrum lighting. That environmental change alone may eliminate some of your tiredness.

Unfortunately, merely changing the kind of lighting you use is no insurance against other environmental causes of tiredness. The high-technology world that has given us many advantages has also given us a chemicals-laden and electromagnetically charged environment that is detrimental to our health. For example, if you live in a smog-bound city like Los Angeles or Cairo, you know how breathing impure, low-oxygen air can make you fatigued. Air pollution is just one of many environmental factors that can lower your energy level. The water that you drink, the pesticides in your food, the stress of overcrowding, the harmful chemicals that waft from synthetic clothing, paint, and even some furniture can all drain your energy.

You can protect yourself to some degree against many of these hazards. You can move to an area with cleaner air. You can filter the air in your car, home, and office. You can buy pure food and water. It just takes more awareness and effort on your part.

HAVE YOU CHECKED WITH MARCUS WELBY? MEDICALLY ORIENTED SOURCES OF TIREDNESS

As we said earlier, in our experience, chronic tiredness is rarely the result of a medical problem. Nevertheless we recommend that you get a thorough physical examination to eliminate the possibility that your tiredness stems from physical illness. Below are brief descriptions of some of the medical causes of tiredness. Please note that this is by no means a comprehensive list.

- *Infections,* whether acute or chronic, can bring on the symptoms of overwhelming exhaustion. They include, but are not limited to, most viral infections, mononucleosis, brain abscess, meningitis, bacterial infections, tuberculosis, parasitic infestations, and osteomyelitis. Two common recently identified diseases that cause extreme fatigue are the Epstein-Barr syndrome and a yeast infection called candida albicans.
- *Anemia.* Most people know that "iron-deficiency anemia" makes one feel run-down, tired. Before you buy iron pills or over-the-counter medicine or tonics, please have your physician check you out. There are several other types of anemia besides that caused by iron-deficiency. All can be diagnosed or ruled out with a simple blood test. Note that anemia is more likely to be a problem for women than for men.
- *Endocrine system problems.* Various kinds of thyroid problems and adult-onset diabetes can cause extreme tiredness.
- *Drug abuse.* The abuse of any intoxicating drug can leave you drained, including alcohol, nicotine, caffeine, barbiturates, and tranquilizers.
- *Cancer.* Fatigue can be an early sign of malignancy.
- *Medication side effects.* Tiredness is often a side effect of such doctor-prescribed medications as sedatives, tranquilizers, antihistamines, anticonvulsants, birth control pills, insulin, and tetracycline. It is also a side effect of vitamins A and D taken in toxic doses.

Sleep disorders. Twenty million people regularly use sleeping pills, even though such pills are only effective in the short run. After you use them for about a week they disturb your normal sleep cycle. Disruptions in your sleep cycle can leave you feeling chronically tired. If sleeplessness or broken sleep is related to a medical problem—e.g., peptic ulcers, asthma, angina, or endocrine disorders—your physician can help. If sleep problems are due to lifestyle habits, the Never Be Tired Again program may be the solution.

THE PSYCHOLOGICAL CAUSES OF TIREDNESS

THE TIREDNESS-STRESS CONNECTION

We are concerned in this book only with the psychological conditions that lead to tiredness and physical ailments. We can categorize all these conditions under the term *stress*—what happens to your body when it feels threatened by some external agency or event. We do not use the word to refer to outside pressure. We define stress as *the body's physiological response* to those pressures; the event that triggers the response is called the "stressor."

Stress, or your biological response to psychological pressures, is a perfectly normal reaction when your life is threatened. It kicks into action automatically and is a superb survival mechanism. In prehistoric times, if you were threatened by a saber-toothed tiger you had to decide instantly whether to stand your ground and fight or run away. In either case you needed an instant surge of energy. We call the mechanism that supplies that energy the fight-or-flight response. Your adrenal glands pour adrenaline into your bloodstream, putting your body's energy system "on alert." Your blood sugar supply increases to deliver the energy for fight or flight. This kind of biochemical reaction is not harmful when it occurs in response to a real-life threatening event.

Problems arise when the fight-or-flight response is continuously and inappropriately triggered by your internal response to non-life-threatening events over a long period of time. The result is chronic tiredness and an increased risk of disease. The adrenal glands, for example, become overtaxed and no longer do their job as well as they should. This situation is critical, for the adrenals have an important role in maintaining your body's well-being beyond their function in the fight-or-flight response. They supply a number of hormones essential to the metabolism of protein, nucleic acids, fat, and carbohydrates. The metabolism of sodium and potassium is also influenced by the adrenal hormonal system. In addition, the adrenal glands secrete hormones that control the immune system response, wound healing, and the integrity of muscles. Damage to or breakdown of the adrenal hormonal system from chronic stress is a serious matter.

SIGNS THAT SIGNAL STRESS

How do you know when you cross the line between moderate stress and severe stress? Here are several clear warning signs that you may be crossing the line.

- *An increased heart rate.* Remember how your heart pounded the first time you asked for a raise or when you asked someone you cared about for a date? Do you get the same reaction now when you face an important business meeting? When a superior criticizes your work? When you have a family quarrel? Then, later, do you feel drained of energy?

- *Pronounced changes in your breathing rate.* Love songs that say "You take my breath away" are quite literally describing the stress response. Do you find it hard to catch your breath when trying to meet a deadline? When the deadline pressure is over, do you feel exhausted?

- *Sweaty palms, perspiration.* The next time you go for a job interview, dry your hands just before you shake hands with the interviewer. Executive recruiters and personnel directors are trained to look for this obvious sign of stress.

- *Sleep disturbances.* Sleeping too much, waking in the middle of the night, or not being able to sleep at all are classic signs of stress.

- *Reduced sex drive.* A lack of libido is a common result of the tiredness that comes from stress. The exercise system we recommend as part of the Never Be Tired Again program increases sex drive. This may be a good reason for you and your partner to embark on the program together.

- *Shivering, trembling.* If you are cold or tremble much of the time with no physical cause, you are probably experiencing a stress response. This symptom is usually followed by an overwhelming desire to sleep.

- *Tense muscles.* Do you continually walk around with a knot in the back of your neck? Are your shoulder blades constantly tense? Do you have lower back problems? Such muscle tension can cause considerable fatigue.
- *Changes in how you perceive things.* Stress can cause blurred vision or affect your psychological perception of the external world. For example, you may sense events happening more slowly than they really are.
- *Increased or decreased ability to concentrate.* Increased ability to concentrate is a common stress symptom. If you have ever gone fishing, you know the feeling when the fish takes the bait—your whole being is focused on that one event. On the negative side, stress can prevent you from being able to concentrate at all. The strain of trying to concentrate under stress is itself fatiguing.
- *Stomach troubles.* Your gastrointestinal tract basically shuts down during stress. You may experience cramps, nausea, and similar symptoms, and you will not get all the energy you should from your food.

SOURCES OF PSYCHOLOGICAL STRESS AND TIREDNESS

It is not necessarily *how many* stressful events are in your life that dictates how stressed you feel. Rather, *it is how much you feel in or out of control of the stress that makes the difference.* If your behavior score in the subtest in chapter 2 is 62 or lower, you may be suffering from stress you feel is out of your control. The main sources of psychological stress and tiredness include the following:

LIFE CHANGES

Everyone experiences stressful events and change. Many are part of normal living—a job change, financial setbacks, the birth of a child, for example. If you are managing your lifestyle well, chances are that you will be able to deal with the ongoing flow of life's changes quite well. If not, you may be in for trouble. The stressful effects of change are cumulative, particularly when many changes occur in a short time. Psychiatrists have studied the kinds of events that cause stress. The death of a spouse, a divorce, a serious illness, marriage, and loss of a job are among the major life changes that can trigger the stress response. If several such changes occur within a short time, stress can intensify sharply.

INTERPERSONAL RELATIONSHIPS

Nothing is more tiring or draining than interpersonal conflict. Joely always asks audiences to list three recent stressful events. Almost without exception the responses involve other people. The most stressful interpersonal problems stem from difficult relationships with people you can't avoid: a spouse, children, parents, in-laws, employers, neighbors. If you are under this kind of interpersonal psychological pressure, or if you scored below 160 on the relationship subtest in chapter 2, you may be running a risk of developing serious illness—a heart attack or ulcers, for example. You are also probably exhausted most of the time. The Never Be Tired Again program will help you deal with the stress by reducing tension and helping to strengthen your immune system. But it is no substitute for a wise counseling program that can help you resolve the root causes of your interpersonal conflicts.

CAREER STRESS

There is the normal fatigue that comes from putting in a good hard day's work, and there is the weary exhaustion that comes from an emotionally stressful day at work. The first kind of tiredness disappears with a good night's sleep. The second lingers, becomes chronic, and may keep you from sleeping. Much work-related stress can stem from relationship problems. Counseling or, if possible, changing to a more satisfying work environment may solve the problem.

Tiredness can also be the result of working under the tyranny of the clock. If you must constantly meet unrealistic and often unachievable deadlines, you are definitely under fatigue-producing stress. David constantly fights his addiction to deadlines. In the past five years he has gradually cured himself of it, but occasionally the tyranny of the clock or calendar gets him down. Joely has given him an ironic prayer to reflect on at such times:

O God, please help me to meet this self-imposed and totally unnecessary deadline!

YOUR ATTITUDES

These, too, can work for or against you. Remember that stress is more than just being temporarily upset about some person or event, more than simply having one or two "bad days" at work. Rather, stress is a recurring, incessant yo-yo process that results in daily wear and tear on your body, constant tiredness, and eventual illness. If you scored below 87 on the Attitude Test in chapter 2, you need to reexamine your feelings and thoughts about yourself and your life. Your internal attitudes may be the real culprit that is making you feel worn out all the time.

The most obvious example of how attitudes can work against you is the sense of overwhelming tiredness that washes over you when you are "bored" by some task. Yet the moment an exciting or challenging opportunity comes along, you are instantly energized! Of course, the relationship between stress, attitudes, and tiredness is not always that clear-cut. You may, for example, harbor an unconscious sense of low self-esteem; therefore, no matter what you do, you believe things won't turn out right. The Never Be Tired Again program can help improve your self-image because you will be charged with new energy and you will look and feel better. However, if low self-esteem or repressed anger, for example, are buried deeply within you, you may want to seek counseling to help defuse these energy-draining feelings.

DEPRESSION AND ANXIETY

Tiredness is the most common symptom of psychological depression. But other symptoms vary by sex and age. Men usually express depression with an attitude of pessimism, guilt, and a sense of helplessness. Women may express their depression, at least in the early stages, with headaches, insomnia, or social withdrawal. (However, remember that depression and/or anxiety may be normal if it occurs as a result of a major tragedy in your life.) The Never Be Tired Again program can help you. Increasingly, the kind of vigorous exercise we recommend is becoming the preferred treatment for depression and/or anxiety, along with professional counseling.

THE BOTTOM LINE ON TIREDNESS

By this time you may be saying to yourself, "This is awfully complicated. Will I ever find the real reason for my tiredness?" You're right. The causes of chronic tiredness are many and often complex. But don't be discouraged. If there proves to be no physical basis for your tiredness, chances are that it has its roots in your lifestyle. If that is the case, the Never Be Tired Again program is the cure.

Chapter 4

Each of Us Is a Living Energy System

If you want to get as much benefit as you possibly can from this book, you will need to forget everything you were taught about the nature of reality.

You will need to go beyond the concept that matter is solid, that you are solid flesh.

You will have to put aside the idea that your body has some sort of internal program that predetermines your physical condition.

THE HUMAN ENERGY SYSTEM

If you want to make exciting changes in your life, you must understand that *you are a living energy system* and that the principles of the science known as quantum physics apply to you just as they do to all other energy systems in the universe.

No doubt you were taught in school that your body is made up of muscles, tissues, cells, blood, and bones. As science became more sophisticated, it learned that every part of the body—as everything in the universe—is made up of atoms which, in turn, are composed of subatomic particles such as electrons, protons, and neutrons. Physicist Fred Alan Wolf has a wonderful description of an atom in his book *Taking the Quantum Leap* (Harper and Row, 1981). If you want to be able to see one of the atoms inside a golf ball, he says, you would have to blow the golf ball up until it was the size of the earth. Then within this earth-sized golf ball an atom would be the size of a golf ball. In order to see the nucleus within that atom, you would have to increase the golf ball–sized atom to the size of a football stadium. The nucleus would then be about the size of a grain of rice within that huge stadium.

Inside this infinitesimal atomic package, enormous electromagnetic energies are stored. Since your body is made up of atoms, it must also be true that every cell in your body is a tiny package filled with that same energy. At the most fundamental level of your being, your body *is* electromagnetic energy. On an electrocardiogram, that energy produces the graph of the pumping vibrations of your heart. Similarly, an electroencephalograph is a representation of the vibrational energy of your brain waves. That each of us is fundamentally a self-contained energy system is a new and exciting finding for Western science. But it is old hat for the East. Chinese medicine has known for centuries that human beings are primarily energy systems, and that balancing the energy fields in each individual is the key to creating a healthy mind and body.

HIGH-ENERGY PHYSICS: BEYOND EINSTEIN

Quantum physics today has some evidence that extends the subatomic world and the electromagnetic concept of energy even farther. Scientists now hypothesize that nature's most fundamental building blocks are "superstrings" of energy, each many billions of degrees smaller than the atom. Simplified, this theory says that the universe and everything in it is a cosmic network of vibrating energy strings. According to Henry Stapp, an eminent physicist from the University of California at Berkeley, we are all linked in "a web of relationships." In other words, Stapp is saying that when you regard the world at the subatomic level, there are only vibrating strings of energy, differing from one another only in the level and condition of vibration. *Thus all energy in the universe is interconnected.*

ENERGY COMMUNICATION

In addition to the evidence for this universal energy linkage, classic experiments in physics lead almost inescapably to the conclusion that *all energy communicates* at the subatomic level.

In a famous experiment, a light is placed in front of a screen with two vertical slits in it. On the other side of the screen is a photographic plate. When light travels through the slits it makes patterns on the photographic plate. When only one slit is open, light striking the plate creates a fuzzy circle in the center of the plate.

What kind of pattern do you think is formed if both slits are open? You might expect that the light would make two circles, or perhaps merge to create a single larger, brighter circle. What actually happens, however, is that the target shows vertical bands of alternating light and darkness, with the lightest band in the center and the darkest at the extreme ends. This does not surprise physicists. They know the bands are the result of a well-known phenomenon called "interference," caused when light particles passing through both slits collide and interfere with one another.

But what happens if we eliminate the interference by changing from continuous light to a "light gun" that fires individual particles of light, called photons. When the gun is fired with only one slit open, the photon makes a bright mark on the photographic plate in a place that was dark when both slits were open and a continuous light source was present.

Now let's open the second slit. Since we are firing individual photons, you might expect the interference would be eliminated. But this is not the case at all. When both slits are open, no bright marks are recorded in the area that was lit when only one slit was open.

How can this be? The question—the central mystery—is put this way by Gary Zukav in his book *The Dancing Wu Li Masters: An Overview of the New Physics* (Bantam Books, 1979): "When we fired our photon and it went through the first slit, how did it 'know' that it could go to an area that must be dark if the other slit were open? In other words, how did the photon know that the other slit was closed?"

Physicists have been forced to conclude that there is some sort of "consciousness" at work—some form of communication between the photons. If we, at our most fundamental level, are made up of superstrings of vibrating energy, it is not illogical to assume that we too, like photons, can "communicate" at this same level with all other forms of energy.

All this may sound like something out of the Twilight Zone. Yet much ongoing research supports the concept. For example, experimenters using biofeedback devices are able to detect changes in a person's blood pressure, skin temperature, muscle tension, and other physical statuses due solely to what that person's brain tells his or her body to do. Using only our thoughts, we can "communicate" with our body to lower or raise skin temperature, dilate or contract blood vessels, reduce or increase muscle tension. In short, we can consciously produce all sorts of measurable changes that once were believed to be uncontrollable physical responses.

A major message of this book is that you can develop this ability yourself. You don't need to be connected to a biofeedback device to learn the techniques. We offer practical and powerful step-by-step high-energy formulas you can begin to use right now to increase your energy, and to enhance the benefits of the Never Be Tired Again program.

To do this, you simply tap into your *energy consciousness.*

DEVELOPING YOUR ENERGY CONSCIOUSNESS

Using quantum physics theory as our model, we define energy consciousness as the sum of all levels of awareness. It includes—but is not limited to—the ego and the id; the unconscious and the subconscious; altered states such as meditative, hypnotic, and trance states; and the higher consciousness. All of these are manifestations, on one level or another, of your energy consciousness.

Your energy consciousness is everywhere. It is in all of your cells and it envelops your body. At the subatomic level, it is connected to the universal web of energy. Moreover, *how well you have developed your energy consciousness directly determines how your life unfolds.* Physicists tell us there is no fixed reality. Rather, what we call reality is a series of probability waves—an infinite number of events that *can* happen. Whatever course your life takes does not occur by chance or accident but is a direct result of your own conscious or unconscious actions. Thus if reality is, as physics now tells us, just a set of probabilities, then what reality becomes for you is determined by the choices you make. You are not just an observer, but a "participant-observer" in your own life.

A choice you make actively and with awareness is a powerful change agent. A choice made passively and without awareness is just as powerful, but rarely is a positive change agent. Whether you like it or not, you are creating your own reality by your choices or nonchoices. You can communicate positive messages to your body, or you can communicate messages of disregard and non-caring. You can choose to be a benevolent participant in your own life or you can choose to abdicate that power. Abdication leads to entropy, another law of physics that says systems tend to decay over time unless something is done to prevent or slow down the decay process. The more conscious choices you make that are beneficial to you as an energy system, the more energy you will have.

MAKE THE QUANTUM LEAP!

Right now we call upon you to make a quantum leap in your own belief system: *Be open to possibilities.*

- Be open to the possibility that you can make profound changes in your health and your energy level by becoming a conscious participant in your own lifestream.
- Be open to the possibility that you can integrate the practical information about nutrition, exercise, dynamic breathing, and visualization that we will provide in subsequent chapters with the explosive power of your own conscious choice, and thus create a healthier and more energetic life for yourself.

THE OXYGEN CONNECTION: THE KEY TO HIGH ENERGY

One of the easiest choices you can make involves oxygen and its effect on your energy level. Oxygen is the most important substance that fuels your body—more important than food, more important than water. *Increasing the amount of oxygen in your system is the key to increasing your energy and never being tired.*

Let's look at how this oxygen-fueled energy-production process works.

The first step your body takes is to convert the food you eat into glucose, amino acids, and fats. The glucose combines with oxygen in your cells and through a further sequence of interactions produces the high-energy molecule *adenosine triphosphate,* or ATP for short. ATP is the real source of the body's energy. If there is insufficient oxygen in your cells, the glucose ferments and produces two molecules of ATP and lactic acid. This is what scientists call an "inelegant" solution to your energy needs, because this process yields only two molecules of ATP. The buildup of lactic acid in the body actually drains energy from your muscles.

In contrast, when there is enough oxygen in your body for all the glucose to combine with it, thirty-six ATP molecules are produced. A great deal more energy is then available to you. Thus, the "elegant" solution—the cleanest and quickest route to a desired result—to increased energy is to get more oxygen into your body.

WHY MOST PEOPLE DO NOT HAVE ENOUGH OXYGEN

But you may ask, "Why wouldn't I have enough oxygen to start with?" After all, everyone breathes. This should mean that everyone has enough oxygen, right? Wrong.

Stress reduces oxygen. When we are stressed we tense our muscles, especially in the upper body. This reduces the blood flow and, since blood carries oxygen, also reduces the oxygen available to cells. Lifestyle habits can also make a big difference. For example, smoking destroys lung tissue, thereby reducing the amount of oxygen a smoker can get with each breath. Not knowing how to breathe properly can decrease the amount of available oxygen. Physical inactivity can lower lung capacity. Eating food that causes a cholesterol buildup in the arteries is still another cause of reduced blood flow. Eating too much salt increases blood pressure and reduces the blood flow. *As you can see, there are any number of reasons why you wouldn't have "enough" oxygen.*

HOW YOU CAN CONSCIOUSLY CHOOSE THE "ELEGANT" SOLUTION FOR ENERGY

If your cells do not get enough oxygen, they have no choice but to convert glucose into lactic acid in order to produce two measly molecules of ATP. If you choose to increase your oxygen supply, you will change reality by allowing your cells the "elegant" alternative. Cardiovascular exercise, for example, increases the amount of oxygen in your bloodstream. By choosing to exercise, you can change the physical reality of your life by giving your cells the opportunity to *produce* more energy.

You can also choose your attitude. Do you see yourself as someone who loves to be active, someone who enjoys the freedom an energized body offers? Or do you see exercise as punishment? Do you see eating high-energy foods as an adventure or as a restriction? These questions may seem like so much verbal fencing, but your attitudes do define reality. The good news is that you can use the techniques of internal programming described in Part III to redefine your reality. You can choose to see yourself getting younger, getting slimmer, increasing your oxygen supply with exercise and high-energy nutrition. You can decide through visualization to see your cells producing more ATP, to see yourself having increased energy, to see yourself never being tired.

Choose to see yourself as you want to be, and that will define your new reality.

QUICK ENERGY CHARGES

The following quick energy charge is the first in a series of ten-minute energy boosters we have placed in appropriate locations throughout this book. You can use them at any time. Most begin with the same five steps. These five steps help you relax and prepare your subconscious mind to receive the specific energy programming statement in step 6. Step 6 is different each time and changes according to the energy message you want your subconscious to absorb. Step 7 brings you back to wakeful reality and is the same for each quick energy charge.

Unlike many people who teach self-programming, we believe there are no hard and fast rules to success. However, we have found that most of our patients prefer the sequencing we recommend in this book. The initial steps are meant to be repetitive so that each time you repeat the process the self-programming is deepened and intensified. You may want to make the quick energy charges into tapes or have someone read them to you slowly until you have learned the steps, but it is not necessary to get them absolutely "right" to benefit. The box below contains the steps that are repeated in the quick energy charges.

THE QUICK ENERGY CHARGE STEPS

Step 1: Getting comfortable

Lie on the floor or sit in a comfortable chair with arm rests. Make certain you won't be disturbed. Pick a time when the house or apartment is quiet. This exercise takes only ten minutes. (It's okay to take longer if you like.)

Step 2: Mind set

Close your eyes and breathe in through your nose slowly and deeply. Fill your stomach first, then your midriff, and then your upper chest. You may want to raise your shoulders slightly to allow even more oxygen to enter your lungs. Hold this breath for a count of four, then exhale slowly through your mouth. As you exhale, feel your shoulders relax and drop, and the muscles in your upper body become less tense and cramped. Say to yourself, "It is all right to give myself this time each day. It is essential that I recharge myself. The more oxygen I take in, the more healthy, vital, and productive I feel."

Step 3: Counting down

Keeping your eyes closed, take a deep breath and exhale slowly. With your mind's eye, scan every muscle in your body. Notice that you are a bit more relaxed than you were before you took that first deep breath. Next, with each long, slow breath, begin counting down from 5 to 1. Inhale as you say "five," exhale as you say "five" again and imagine yourself going down a flight of stairs. Continue counting down through 1. Notice that with each breath and each stair you are more relaxed than you were before. After you have taken the five breaths and are at the bottom of the stairs, see yourself walking through a beautiful forest—lush, green, warm, inviting. Walk toward a crystal-clear pond and lie on the soft grass next to it. See yourself completely alone, secure, and totally relaxed. Feel the sun shining on you, keeping you snug and warm.

Step 4: Deepening the memory

Pay attention to what it feels like to be alert and relaxed at the same time. Say to yourself, "Each time I count from five to one, I reach a more profound, relaxed, and creative level of mind than the last time I entered this level of consciousness."

Step 5: Sensing your internal energy

Now, breathing normally, pay attention to the sound and sensations of your body. Remember that your body, as an energy system, is made up of a large network of vibrating strings of energy. Allow those strings to vibrate in harmony with one another. Feel the oneness that comes from this recognition. If other thoughts come into your mind, pretend you are simply an observer of your body. Let those thoughts pass through your head without judgment. Continue to focus on the vibrations of your energy strings.

Step 6: Energy programming

Each quick energy charge has an individualized programming statement for Step 6.

Step 7: Reentry

When you're ready, go back to the stairs. Count from 1 to 5 as you go up to the stairs. When you reach the top stair, open your eyes slowly, take a moment to reorient yourself, and then go about your day feeling more relaxed and more energetic.

QUICK ENERGY CHARGE #1

A Getting Started Daydream

Steps 1–5: See above.

Step 6: Energy Programming

Breathing slowly and deeply, see the oxygen entering every cell in your body. See your tiredness and tension melting into the grass, leaving you relaxed and alert. With each breath, breathe in increased energy and breathe out tiredness and stress. See the energy come into your body as pure white light.

Now that your deepest self is tuned in and harmonizing in this relaxed but alert state, imagine yourself the way you want to be. Look at yourself in the mirror of your mind and continue to gaze at the You that you have always wanted to be. Say to yourself, "I am going to write and direct a play in which I will star as the real Me. It will be a great success because there is nothing I cannot do with my life." Know that you can use all the techniques in this book to make this a prize-winning play. See your family and friends making up the audience. Hear them applaud each movement, each decision, each change you make in your lifestyle. Look into the audience and sense the awe and admiration each person has for you. Listen to the roar of a standing ovation and know it is happening to you now.

Step 7: See box above.

Chapter 5

Too Tired for Sex?

The Price of Success

Larry had everything. After fifteen years of fourteen-hour workdays, he owned a thriving business, an elaborate home in the best neighborhood, a collection of vintage automobiles, a summer cottage on a lake, and money to burn. Why, then, did his wife of twenty-five years desert him recently for another man, leaving behind her mink coat and a Mercedes?

Ignore all the excuses she made and the reasons she gave. Larry's wife left him because he was almost always too tired to make love to her. And why was he too tired for sex? Because he was so involved in his business that he neglected to take care of himself. As the result of this unbalanced lifestyle, Larry had lots of pressures along with business. He had high blood pressure; serious addictions to cigarettes, fatty foods, and chocolate bars. He was also addicted to his own adrenaline, so that by the end of the day he came home exhausted and hungry. He ate his dinner in front of the TV set and usually fell asleep in his chair. Obviously the issue of "sex" never came up. Larry was much too tired for that!

With today's emphasis on career success, chances are that tiredness is taking the joy out of sex for many men and women. Like Larry, many of us are so exhausted by evening that the only thing we want to do in bed is sleep. Lack of sexual energy and even sexual interest is a common complaint. The *New York Post* recently surveyed a cross-section of American women, most of whom were between eighteen and thirty-five—young women—about their sexual activity. Fifty-six percent said they didn't make love as often as they would like to, and 54 percent said that fatigue was the main reason they didn't want to make love. Psychologist William B. Flynn, Jr., director of the Merrimack Valley Counseling Association in Nashua, New Hampshire, and a specialist in marriage, family, and sex therapy, says that 45 percent of his clients, male and female, claim to be chronically tired. As a result they have difficulty functioning sexually.

Why are you too tired for sex?

As we noted in chapter 3, the reasons you are tired all the time run the gamut from physical factors to psychological blocks to a counterproductive lifestyle. Whatever the cause, however, the upshot can be that you're just too tired for sex. The results are predictably unhappy: Both your self-esteem and your sense of masculinity or femininity suffer; there is a great loss of intimacy with your spouse or lover, and because this intimacy is one of the foundations of your personal and family relationships, these relationships can be severely weakened. Far from least is the fact that you are depriving yourself of one of life's most rewarding pleasures.

TOO TIRED FOR SEX: THE PHYSICAL FACTORS

SMOKING

The medical community has known for years that smoking constricts blood vessels. Now researchers are discovering that the negative effects of smoking are evident in the small arteries of the penis, reducing the ability to have an erection. As the narrow penile arteries become more constricted, less blood is able to flow into the penis. This means that a man's erection may become weaker over time. When smoking is combined with other diseases that affect the arteries (arteriosclerosis, diabetes, hypertension, high cholesterol), the incidence of impotence—and, of course, tiredness—increases dramatically. Sperm abnormalities have also been reported among long-time or heavy cigarette smokers.

Although research on the link between smoking and reduced sexual functioning has so far been limited to men, it is not unrealistic to assume that smoking has a similar effect on women's sexual capacity. Constricted blood vessels will not inhibit a woman's ability to perform sexually in the same way they inhibit male performance, but it is reasonable to assume that decreased flow of blood to a woman's sexual organs diminishes sensation. During sexual excitement, a woman's blood rushes to engorge her breasts, clitoris, and vagina. This adds to sexual tension and therefore to sexual feelings. If constricted blood vessels impede this flow, we believe it could have a negative impact on the intensity of a woman's sensory responses.

ARTERIAL DAMAGE

Diabetes, hypertension, and elevated cholesterol and/or triglyceride levels also tend to narrow the arteries and reduce the flow of blood to the sexual organs, resulting in impaired erection and reduced sensation. Doctors at the Center for Study and Research on Impotence in Paris studied the effect of these arterial risk factors by comparing 440 impotent men with potent men of the same age. According to their report in the British medical journal *Lancet,* blood pressure in the penile arteries was significantly lower when two or more of the risk factors were present. If three risk factors were present, there was a 100 percent likelihood that the man would be organically impotent—unable to have an erection because of physical damage. (Inorganic impotence occurs when a man is physically able to have an erection during sleep and perhaps on awakening but for psychological reasons is unable to achieve or sustain an erection while making love to his partner.)

CANDIDA: A REAL TURN-OFF

Tiredness in and of itself is enough to put a damper on sexual desire, but candidiasis—a chronic yeast infection—has an even greater impact on libido. Fatigue is one of its symptoms.

According to Dr. Richard Noble, a specialist in the management of candidiasis who practices in Cardiff by the Sea in southern California, chronic infection with candida albicans yeast can cause a wide range of physical, neurological, and psychological symptoms. Obviously vaginal irritation will inhibit a woman's sexual interest and response, but that symptom is not the only potential cause of a decrease in her libido. Dr. Noble cites research done in Japan indicating that candidiasis also affects the functioning of various endocrine systems, including those that regulate sex hormones. The yeast infection seems to block the receptor sites for the hormones and interferes with the reception of the message of sexual arousal in the sexual organs. Over time, a person suffering from chronic candidiasis may cease to feel arousal. This problem coupled with the extreme tiredness that often accompanies candidiasis severely reduces the chances for a fulfilling sex life.

OBESITY

Obesity is a two-edged sword in terms of sexuality. It has both physical and psychological ramifications. Physically, obesity makes you tired. It puts a serious strain on the cardiovascular system because the heart must pump blood through a much larger network of veins and arteries. The rest of your organs are similarly taxed when you're carrying around too much weight.

Obesity is equally devastating from a psychological perspective. It's hard to *feel* sexy when you don't think you *look* sexy. Many obese men and women don't want to make love because they don't feel attractive or sexy. Some lay a guilt-punishment trip on themselves: "Since I can't control my compulsive eating, I'm 'bad'," they tell themselves. Believing that, they assume that they do not deserve sexual pleasure and repress their desires.

Obesity is medically defined as being 20 percent over the normal weight for your age, sex, and height. Many people who have a poor body image are not clinically obese, even though they weigh more than they would like to.

DIET

Your favorite food could be ruining your sex life.

A Romantic Evening?

Friday night. Thank heaven. Just the two of you. Your favorite restaurant. Gourmet food. Superb wine. Lavish desserts. Candlelight. Violins. Visions of a romantic evening at home after dinner.

Two hours later the scene shifts. Driving home, you're logy, your senses dulled. You open the car windows to stay awake. Once home you can hardly make it up the stairs. You both collapse into bed and promptly fall asleep. Another romantic evening down the drain!

This scenario is not atypical. As we noted previously, not all of your favorite food is energy-producing. In fact, many people have either food allergies or food sensitivities that can cause extreme tiredness, bloating, indigestion, headaches, rashes, and flatulence. None of these conditions is conducive to a happy sex life.

If the scene above has happened to you, there's a good chance you are sensitive to certain foods, and more than likely those foods are your favorites. Moreover, you probably had a high-fat, high-sugar, high-protein meal with little or no complex carbohydrate. Your body has to work especially hard to digest the fat and protein, leaving little energy for anything else, let alone sex. In addition, the refined sugar you ate triggers the stress response, creating a short-lived high followed by a rapid bottoming-out of your blood sugar. The short-term result is overwhelming tiredness. When the choice is between gourmet dining and romance, we'll take romance!

DRUGS, BOOZE, AND SEX

If you expect to have an active sex life, don't buy into the myth that drugs and/or alcohol will enhance your sexual performance. Quite the opposite is true.

Large amounts of alcohol depress the central nervous system and inhibit sexual desire. The initial post-drink feeling of increased sexual desire stems from the lowered anxiety produced by a small amount of alcohol. But this effect is short-lived. In the final analysis, alcohol suppresses the neurologic sexual reflex pathways.

Besides alcohol, the drugs that adversely affect sexual functioning include amphetamines, barbiturates, cocaine, marijuana, and heroin. In addition, many drugs that you may take for "medicinal purposes" or that are prescribed by your physician can lead to exhaustion and/or impotence. For example, antihypertensive drugs, antihistamines, tranquilizers, and other psychopharmacological drugs are leading causes of impotence and depressed sexual functioning. Living the Never Be Tired Again lifestyle can be an effective substitute for drug therapy. Ask your physician to help you—perhaps you can lower your blood pressure with diet, exercise and relaxation techniques rather than with drugs. The payoff will be improved sexual functioning. If you truly want to keep romance in your life, avoid drugs whenever possible. If you must drink, limit yourself to one glass of wine when you expect a romantic end to your evening.

TOO TIRED FOR SEX: PSYCHOLOGICAL FACTORS

ATTITUDES AND MYTHS ABOUT SEX

Can you visualize a couple in their twenties making love? Of course you can. How about a couple in their forties? Fifties? Seventies? Eighties? If you feel uncomfortable with the images of increasingly older couples making love, you have fallen victim to a major self-defeating myth—the myth that sexual desire and ability disappear as we age.

There is no automatic age limit for sexual interest and functioning for either men or women! Men who are only reasonably healthy can function sexually into their eighties and nineties. We believe that for men who live a Never Be Tired Again lifestyle there is no upper limit at all.

A young man will reach a full erection within three to five seconds of mental or physical stimulation. A man in his fifties to seventies may need two to three times as long. On the face of it that doesn't sound good. But do a little arithmetic and you'll find a fifty- to seventy-year-old man requires only six to fifteen seconds to achieve an erection. Older men also have a distinct and often overlooked sexual advantage. Young men tend to climax quickly; older men are able to maintain an erection for a longer time before ejaculation. There is a lot to be said for age and experience! According to Dr. William Masters, the best guarantee of being able to make love as you get older is good health, an interested and interesting partner, and continued sexual activity.

DEPRESSION

Depression can take much of the sexual joy out of life. Depending on which study you read, 51 to 73 percent of depressed people report a loss of sexual interest—coupled with such other symptoms of depression as extreme tiredness, low energy level, irritability, anxiety, low self-esteem, and a desire to withdraw from others—which often leads to conflict between the depressed person and his or her partner. Divorced men and women often say depression and its attendant problems were important contributing factors to the breakup of their marriage.

TOO STRESSED FOR SEX?

One sign of excessive stress is a reduced sex drive, no doubt as a result of the sleep disturbances and fatigue associated with stress.

A relationship that isn't working can drain sexual energy. Picture a couple having a fight over spending habits. Hear the shouting, the hurled accusations; flinch as the door is slammed. Now imagine the couple making up and starting to make love. Is the picture getting hazy? Of course it is . . . the ending doesn't usually happen that way.

There are some couples who find sex more exciting after a good fight. For most people, however, anger—especially repressed anger—is a great inhibitor of sexual desire. Expressed anger can be dealt with. Unexpressed anger and resentment have far more devastating effects on a relationship.

When your partner is too tired to make love, are you secretly relieved? Is your initial inner response to a sexual overture one of annoyance? Do you find reasons not to engage in your partner's favorite sexual caresses or positions? These are common signs of repressed anger. Repressed anger and resentment are like termites; they eat away at the foundation of your relationship.

WHAT ABOUT "REAL TIREDNESS"?

"For heaven's sake," you mutter, "can't I be just too pooped for pleasure once in a while?" Sure you can. Fatigue is not always the result of illness, nor does it always have to be psychological in nature. Sometimes you can get tired from a heavy work load. Sometimes you *can* be too tired for sex.

Fatigue that saps sexual interest is a common complaint of two-career couples who must juggle two jobs, children, social obligations, and personal space. Under these conditions something has to give; often it is their sex life that suffers.

Charles Reilly, a Newton, Massachusetts, psychologist and an instructor in psychiatry at Harvard Medical School, says upper middle class, two-career couples often feel their sex life is not spontaneous enough, that they have lost the sense of fun and playful joy that once marked their relationship. To remedy the situation, he suggests couples learn to schedule spontaneity!

This means learning to get balance in your life. If you find that you are chronically too tired for sex, you need to schedule time for sex. For example, some of our friends regularly arrange romantic weekends at a nearby hotel or motel. They either exchange child-care with friends or hire a sitter. You can schedule one evening a week on a similar basis for a romantic interlude—at home or at a favorite love nest. Maintaining your sex life despite the fatiguing pressures of daily life requires good management of precious time and the establishment of priorities.

STEPS YOU CAN TAKE TO GET MORE ENERGY FOR SEX

If you find you are too tired for sex most of the time, there are steps you can take to change the situation.

Make an appointment for a physical examination. Don't be afraid or ashamed to mention your decreased sex drive to your physician. He or she can help identify and treat possible physical factors contributing to your problem and may suggest lifestyle changes to help you control or correct whatever illnesses or poor habits are proving sexual downers for you.

If you feel your lack of interest in sex is due to a breakdown in your relationship or to sexual problems from your past, *get professional help.* Says San Diego psychotherapist Penelope Young, "No one needs to feel they cannot have a great relationship and great sex. We are fortunate today because we understand the dynamics of healthy relationships, and know what it takes to make them work. We can teach people to communicate more effectively, and help them learn how to resolve differences. We also have an improved knowledge of sexual technology. For women, there are simple techniques to increase orgasmic capacity; for men, simple procedures to prevent premature ejaculation."

Change the lifestyle habits that lead to your feeling chronically tired.

Get yourself into shape physically. Increase your energy. Improve your ability to handle stress, and change your outlook on life!

How can the Never Be Tired Again program help? By addressing the major causes of tiredness in a no-nonsense way. The nutritional program's high-energy recipes help control weight, cholesterol level, and blood pressure. The exercise program helps fight depression and increases your ability to deal with everyday stress. The quick energy charges not only help you combat daily waves of tiredness, they also help you improve your self-image and project that improved self-image to others.

Unless you have a serious medical or psychological problem, making the appropriate lifestyle changes will create the high energy that you need and want for a fulfilling sex life.

Chapter 6

Food, Love, and Energy

We play a word association game with the participants in our workshops. We ask them to call out words that describe what food represents to them. Most often we hear such words as *security, guilt, comfort, energy, reward.* Invariably the group votes that the meaning of food can be summed up in one word: *love.*

A Sad but True American Love Story

John B. first had problems with high blood pressure in his early thirties. Medication reduced his pressure almost to normal, but the side effects of the antihypertensive drug made him tired most of the time. It also made him impotent. Eventually John got so fatigued and so depressed he seldom was up to taking his wife, Sally, out for dinner or an evening's entertainment. John's doctor told him that he was working too hard and to take some time off. He didn't. . . .

Over a period of years John's marriage withered away. Sally, not surprisingly, came to feel totally neglected and sexually unfulfilled. Every night after dinner John fell asleep exhausted. Some nights he was even too tired to climb the stairs to the bedroom. On those nights he slept in the chair in front of the TV. With intimacy of any kind gone from the marriage, Sally got a divorce (and a new, more energetic husband).

To allay his deepening feelings of inadequacy, John began to fill up on fatty foods and sweets. Within a year his cholesterol level was over 300, and he suffered a severe heart attack. Later he had to undergo open heart surgery. The day he was released from the hospital John cheered himself up with a thick shake and a double cheeseburger at his favorite fast food place!

John really knows where love comes from, doesn't he?

THE PSYCHOLOGY OF FOOD AND LOVE

In our Never Be Tired Again vocabulary, *diet* is a dirty word, a word that often elicits feelings of guilt, resentment, and frustration. Your emotional feelings about food and need for oral gratification through food began the moment you were born. As you nursed or drank your bottle, food and feelings of love, security, trust, sensory pleasure, and gratification became inextricably linked. No wonder the word *diet* implies deprivation, even actual or emotional starvation, to many people.

As a child, most of us were rewarded for good behavior with special food treats. We were also punished for bad behavior by having our favorite food treats taken away for a time. This reward-punishment syndrome strengthened and reinforced our emotional attachment to certain foods. (In adult life, that attachment is reinforced by the media. Consider: For every dollar spent on health research in this country, over $100 is spent to advertise food.)

As you grew up, you learned to associate food and the rituals of food with pleasurable social functions, and often with religious observances. The food customs you learned took on emotional overtones as well. For example, caviar is considered "sophisticated" adult food. Peanut butter and jelly bring back pleasant memories of growing up. "Quiet little dinners for two" are reminiscent of romance and sex. Some foods, like certain mushrooms, are said to have magical properties. In some religious and cultural groups certain foods are taboo. Pork, for example, is forbidden to Muslims and Jews. Mormons may not drink alcohol or caffeine. Food is even sexually stereotyped: Steak and potatoes are considered a man's meal, while cucumber sandwiches are deemed appropriate for a ladies' garden party.

What does all this mean? Simply that it's not easy to modify your eating patterns even when there is a life-threatening reason to do so, because the process involves your deepest feelings about love, security, social status, trust, and other powerful behavioral motivators. Fortunately, since eating habits are a learned behavior, they can be modified by the same methods that are used to change any learned behavior.

LEARNING TO LOVE HIGH-ENERGY FOODS

Although our eating modification program is geared toward gaining more energy and better health rather than toward losing weight, your weight will normalize on this program. You will lose weight without counting calories or going hungry. But there is a trade-off: You must teach yourself to stay within our guidelines.

Here are ten easy-to-follow steps that will help you make permanent modifications in your eating habits:

1. Set specific, long-term nutritional goals.

Psychologists have long been studying the relationship between goal-setting and performance. Repeated studies show that men and women who have a sense of responsibility and control over their lives do better at almost everything—school, work, interpersonal relationships. One of the best ways to reinforce this aspect of one's personality is to set highly specific goals and objectives and make sure they can be measured. That is the key to successful goal-setting.

Example of a poorly stated goal:

● I will improve my eating habits.

Example of a long-term, measurable nutritional goal:

● Three months from today I will no longer drink caffeinated coffee.

2. Break your long-term nutritional goals down into short-term goals you can achieve right away.

Examples:

● I will buy some water-processed decaffeinated coffee today. (If you like to grind your own coffee, buy decaffeinated coffee beans.)

● Tonight I will mix three parts of the regular coffee to one part of the decaffeinated coffee and keep it in a special jar.

● Every three weeks, I'll increase the amount of the decaffeinated coffee in the mix until it is 100 percent decaffeinated.

● I will plan some way to get decaffeinated coffee at work. (This may involve buying a single-cup coffee dripper.)

Psychologically, the problem with abruptly eliminating some foods from your diet is that doing so can leave a real social or emotional gap in your life. For instance, some people use the traditional coffee break as a time to relax. Going out for a drink after work is an opportunity to socialize with office colleagues. If you cut out dessert, how are you going to feel rewarded after your hard day at work? If you eliminate these things without finding a replacement, you'll probably feel deprived, angry, or upset.

The trick is to find acceptable substitutes. For example, water-processed decaffeinated coffee doesn't contain the harmful ingredients of chemically processed decaffeinated coffee, and it tastes the same as regular coffee. When you grind water-processed coffee beans, they smell delicious. Try herb teas. Hot water with lemon is surprisingly tasty. Instead of an alcoholic drink, order a Virgin Mary (a Bloody Mary without vodka) or bubbly mineral water and fresh lime. Don't give up desserts altogether. Make an effort to find acceptable alternatives, such as baked apples without sugar, or fresh strawberries, or air-popped popcorn.

3. Reward your achievement immediately with something you like.

Decide in advance what reward you will give yourself when you achieve your goal. This may seem to be an unnecessary step, but that's only because you are looking at it from the viewpoint of the rational adult side of your personality. The child inside us all not only likes but needs reinforcement. That child will resist making changes unless you can show that working toward your goal will be fun—and rewards are part of the fun. You don't have to choose an expensive reward but it does have to be something you enjoy.

Appropriate rewards:

- A chance to read a book you've been wanting to read for a long time. Take time out just to read for pleasure.
- Go to the movies on impulse.
- Get a professional manicure.
- Pay someone else to shovel snow or mow the lawn next time that has to be done.

4. Make certain the reward does not conflict with good eating habits.

Example of a conflicting reward:

- A hot fudge sundae

Examples of appropriate rewards:

- A baked apple with cinnamon
- A new murder mystery to read
- A new low-fat cookbook

You must pick the reward yourself. The rewards someone else would choose for you may be motivating to them, but not to you.

5. Change the scene of your poor eating habits.

Example:
- Don't allow yourself to snack in front of the television or in the bedroom. Allow yourself to eat only in the dining area.

6. *Challenge yourself to eat high-energy foods.*
Examples:
- Throw out all the high-fat and high-sugar snacks in the house.
- Make a trip to the grocery store (or a good health food store if one is near) to buy healthy snacks. Be willing to be adventurous.

7. *Involve your loved ones in your high-energy eating program.*
Examples:
- Ask your spouse to work with you in planning a timetable for gradually eliminating sugar from the family diet.
- Ask a friend to caution you (gently and quietly) every time you eat candy.

8. *Evaluate and reevaluate your progress.*
Each time you slip back into an old energy-draining eating habit, talk to yourself and others about it. For example, if you backslide and eat a candy bar, don't lay an emotional trip on yourself. Instead, figure out how to avoid the situation that triggered your relapse. Try buying your newspaper at a newsstand that doesn't display candy bars up front. Bring some fruit to work to eat during your mid-morning and mid-afternoon slumps. If you eat when you're tired or upset, have special treats on hand (like the desserts in our seven-day program).

9. *Learn to eat high-energy foods from someone who has already done it.*
Join a health club. Look for new friends who have successfully mastered the art of high-energy living. We are all social animals and tend to mimic those with whom we associate. Read about men and women who have overcome serious health problems and have subsequently become vibrant and active through good nutrition and exercise. A list of some of our favorite magazines is at the end of this book.

10. *Keep yourself stimulated to improve.*
For an effective daily reminder of the transformation you are undertaking, post one list of your nutritional goals over your desk and another on your bathroom mirror. Keep your goals in front

of you at all times. Cross them off the list as you successfully complete them.

ENERGY, FOOD, AND LOVE GO TOGETHER

As we mentioned earlier, modifying your eating habits means changing some of your feelings about food. This translates into having to deal with some of your most powerful emotions, particularly your need for love and security.

When we first began to switch to a high-energy nutritional program, we found ourselves constantly slipping back into our old "feeling loved is eating certain foods" habits. One of our favorite ways to express self-love was to use ice cream as a reward for a hard day's work. After a little self-observation, we realized we could not resist raiding the refrigerator for ice cream when we were under stress. So one of the ways we prevented backsliding was simply not to have ice cream, chips, and other irresistible goodies in our kitchen. If they were not in the cupboard or the refrigerator we *couldn't* eat them—it was a physical impossibility!

If you make sure that you have healthy and tasty snacks around, neither you nor your family should feel deprived. Keep your favorite fruit in the house even if you feel it's an extravagance. After all, how many times have you paid several dollars for gourmet ice cream without thinking twice? How many times have you spent a lot of money for liquor without batting an eyelash? Yet, how many times have you balked at paying three dollars or more for fresh raspberries, even though they are your favorite fruit? Think about the games we play with ourselves over what we will spend money on and what we won't allow ourselves to buy. Start loving yourself more; allow yourself to indulge in healthy treats.

Learn to prepare your food in healthy ways that taste good. The key is tasting good. If you don't like the way your food tastes, you won't eat it even if you know it's good for you. We have learned a trick you may find helpful. When we try a new recipe we make sure to include in the rest of the meal something we especially like. If the new recipe is a total loser, at least we won't be left feeling hungry or emotionally deprived. It's especially important to use this approach with children. You'll find a creative challenge in discovering food that tastes good and working out gourmet ways to enhance its flavor.

To get the most energy from your food, you must prepare it in ways that conserve nutrients. Learn to steam food lightly rather than boil it. Learn to eat a lot of raw food—salads without oil-based dressings, fruit, carrot sticks. Finally, learn to eat your food in the nutritionally correct order. High-protein foods such as fish and tofu should be eaten first. Then eat faster-moving foods such as grains, steamed greens, raw vegetables, and fruits so they help push the slower-moving proteins through your digestive system more quickly.

QUICK ENERGY CHARGE #2

Food and Love

Steps 1–5: See the instructions preceding Quick Energy Charge #1 in chapter 4.

Step 6: Energy programming

Breathing slowly and deeply, see the oxygen entering every cell in your body. See your tiredness and tension melting into the grass, leaving you relaxed and alert. With each breath, breathe in increased energy and breathe out tiredness and stress. See the energy come into your body as pure white light.

Now that your deepest self is tuned in and harmonizing in this relaxed but alert state, imagine yourself walking through a beautiful vegetable garden. Notice the beauty in the design, the colors, the shape of each plant and flower. Pick your favorite vegetable. Touch its surface gently. Hold it in your hand and feel the sensation of your palm against its skin. Put it down and continue your walk.

Go to the part of the garden that contains the orchard. Look at the rainbow of colors represented by the many fruits that grow here. Inhale the sweet incense of the blossoms. Pick your favorite fruit. Take a bite. Inhale its flavor and sweetness.

Now, as you continue to walk through the garden and orchard, sense the energy vibrations coming from the plants and trees. Sit down under the shade of your favorite apple tree. Feel at peace, knowing that all the vegetables and fruits growing here are part of the wonderful, creative universal energy system. Know that they are designed to nourish you and that ultimately they will become one with your own energy cells.

Step 7: Reentry. See the instructions preceding Quick Energy Charge #1 in chapter 4.

Part II

THE NEVER BE TIRED AGAIN NUTRITION PROGRAM

Chapter 7

High-Energy Nutrition Can Reduce Both Weight and Cholesterol

You Can Eat Your Muffins and Lose Weight, Too!
Alex's Story

"It would be nice to lose a little weight, but I'm more concerned about my cholesterol," Alex said during our initial discussion. "I've been going to a heart specialist for a year. He's put me on powdered drinks to help me lose weight, but I've actually gained a couple of pounds the past year. My cholesterol level is 260, well above the normal range. He says that it's genetic, and I'll never get it below 220."

Alex also suffered such severe allergies that he had to hire a full-time chauffeur: "My allergy medication makes me so drowsy that I'd fall asleep behind the wheel and kill myself," he said. "I always thought of myself as a high-energy person, but over the last few years it takes more effort to do the things I need to do. And then there is hardly any energy left to do the things I want to do."

Since in our program the average client's cholesterol level drops 15 percent in seven days, we felt comfortable telling Alex that he could expect to lower his cholesterol about that much. We also assured him he would lose weight and get a new infusion of energy.

In terms of weight control, we teach that calories don't count. "If you eat the right kinds of food you don't need to be concerned about counting calories," we told Alex. He took us at our word. But as we watched Alex during his week in our program, we began to fear he might prove to be the exception to the rule. He ate everything in sight and even ordered extra food.

He did, however, follow all of our nutritional guidelines for reducing cholesterol and took part fully in the exercise program. One week into the program, the group had follow-up blood tests done and measurements taken. Alex shook his head. "I lost an inch and three-quarters from my midriff and waist. I never would have believed it!"

When the results of the blood tests came in. Alex's cholesterol had dropped 30 percent, from 260 to 182. As an added gift, he had stopped taking his allergy medication midweek and had so much energy he talked about adding extra exercise sessions (which we vetoed).

A month after the program ended, Alex told us he had lost another six pounds despite continuing to eat large amounts of food. "My energy level is phenomenal," he reported. "I'm in and out of planes all the time. My schedule has been crazy, but I'm able to work longer and harder than I ever thought possible."

Alex checks in with us once a month or so. He's still losing weight slowly and steadily. His cholesterol has dropped even lower, to 176. This means platelets are no longer building up on his arterial walls. He's still off his allergy medication and he says performance "in and out of bed gets better and better."

PROGRAM READINESS TEST

Answer these three questions "yes" or "no."
1. Are you interested in maintaining a normal weight level without dieting?
2. Are you interested in a nutritional program that encourages you to eat between meals?
3. If you need to lose weight, would you like to do so without feeling hungry?

We ask these questions of everyone who enters our program. Needless to say, there are a lot more "yes" than "no" answers! If you answered "yes" to any of the questions, or if you would simply like to increase your energy, read on.

THE FIVE RULES OF HIGH-ENERGY NUTRITION

There are only five rules you must follow if you want to have the benefits of high-energy nutrition. They are:
1. No more than 20 percent of your calories should come from fat.
2. No more than 10 percent of your calories should come from animal protein.
3. Make sure your food contains no additives, preservatives, or refined products. This includes white sugar, white flour, and white rice.
4. Eat a wide variety of foods.

5. Include cardiovascular exercise in your schedule at least four days a week for cardiovascular fitness, and at least five days a week if you want to lose weight.

If you follow these rules you won't need to be concerned about counting the calories you eat. The number of calories you eat is not as important as the kinds and quality of the food you eat. Alex's story illustrates what is possible. You can get similar results for yourself. In the chapters in this section we will explain in detail how to follow each of our rules. Be open to:

- The possibility that you'll love this new way of eating
- The possibility that the rules will be easy to follow and easy to stick with
- The possibility that you will be healthier, happier, and more energized than you ever have been

Focus on these possibilities when you talk to yourself in your internal programming sessions—and when you talk to other people. Make choices that support *you* and the changes you want to make in your life.

QUICK ENERGY CHARGE #3

Opening the Door to Energy

Steps 1–5: See the instructions preceding Quick Energy Charge #1 in chapter 4.

Step 6: Energy programming

Breathing slowly and deeply, see the oxygen entering every cell in your body. See your tiredness and tension melting into the grass, leaving you relaxed and alert. With each breath, breathe in increased energy and breathe out tiredness and stress. See the energy come into your body as pure white light.

Now that your deepest self is tuned in and harmonizing in this relaxed but alert state, imagine yourself walking toward a large, beautiful marble building in the middle of the forest. Walk up to the front door and look at the engraved brass door marker. Notice that it reads "Unlimited Possibility Entrance."

Pause a moment. Think about what it would be like to grow healthier with each passing day, what it would be like to have boundless energy and vitality. Imagine yourself eating new and wonderful gourmet food that provides your body with delicious nourishment. See yourself reaching your ideal state of physical fitness and health.

Now step through the door. Walk through this marvelous building of unlimited possibilities. Open yourself to them. Imprint them on your mind and your heart as you stroll back outside into the forest and head toward your reentry stairs.

Step 7: Reentry. See the instructions preceding Quick Energy Charge #1 in chapter 4.

Chapter 8

The Fat/Energy Connection

Unless you have just arrived from Mars, you know you should cut down on dietary fat. But do you *really* know why? Would you like to know how?

In this chapter you will learn:

- Why fat is so fattening
- How to implement the Never Be Tired Again 20 percent fat rule
- Why you don't need to count calories ever again
- The ill-starred relationship between fat and energy
- How the fat/cholesterol connection works
- Which foods are high in fat
- A quick and easy way to figure out exactly how much fat is in the foods you buy
- How to choose delicious nonfattening substitutes for fatty foods

WHY CUT DOWN ON FAT?

According to the American Medical Association, dietary fat is one of the main contributing factors in heart disease and cancer. AMA guidelines say that no more than 30 percent of the calories you eat should be fat. We believe that even this percentage is too high. Medical research shows that there is no real difference in breast, colon, and rectal cancer rates within the 30 to 45 percent fat range. Not until the fat content of a diet drops to 20 percent do significantly lower cancer rates show up.

Using this concept of percent of calories derived from fat is a much healthier way to assess the value of your diet than simply counting total calories. In experiments, rats fed low-calorie but proportionately high-fat diets still had a high percentage of fat-developed cancers. The fat/cancer connection has been seen in humans, too. Dr. Piero Dolara, of the University of Florence, noted in the July 1987 *New England Journal of Medicine* that the traditional Mediterranean diet—pasta and bread plus moderate amounts of meat and dairy products—has changed drastically in recent years. From 1910 to 1980 meat consumption increased five-fold and the consumption of total fats tripled. According to Dr. Dolara, the incidence of colon and breast cancer increased significantly as the percentage of fat in the Italian diet rose.

FORGET ABOUT CALORIES!

We have three excellent reasons for making that statement:
- First, calorie counts tell you nothing about the *quality* of your food.
- Second, calories tell you nothing about the total amount of *fat* you are consuming.
- Third, counting calories makes you crazy.

We have a much more effective way to control the amount of fat in your diet. It's simple: *Don't eat anything that derives more than 20 percent of its calories from fat.* Later in this chapter we will list high-fat foods you should avoid in order to meet the 20 percent rule.

If you never eat any food that has more than 20 percent fat—and if you follow the rule about protein spelled out in chapter 9—*you will never have to count another calorie as long as you live.*
- You will be able to maintain a normal weight.
- You will never be hungry because you will be able to eat satisfying meals and snack when you want.
- You will be using nutrition to increase rather than drain your energy.

Does following the 20 percent fat rule mean you can never again eat any food on the high-fat list? No, it doesn't. But if you choose to eat high-fat foods then you *will* need to count calories so that the fat in your overall diet doesn't account for more than 20 percent of your total caloric intake.

WHY FAT IS SO FATTENING

Fat is an astonishing 225 percent more fattening than carbohydrate or protein! Orthodox nutritional knowledge says fat is worth 9 calories a gram. In comparison, carbohydrate and protein are each worth 4 calories a gram. But more recent research by Harvard University expert Dr. Mark Hegsted suggests that fat is actually worth 11 calories a gram. He says traditional nutritionists arrived at the 9-calories-a-gram figure by measuring the amount of heat produced by fat in a laboratory setting with laboratory equipment. He claims that the body is more efficient at using fat than lab machines indicate, and other research supports his findings.

Moreover, when you eat fat your body doesn't have to work as hard to metabolize it as it does when you eat carbohydrates. For example, your body uses only 3 percent of the calories in fat to do the job of processing and storing it. This means that for every 100 calories of fat you eat, your body can store 97 calories. In contrast, when you eat carbohydrates in the form of vegetables, whole grains, and the like, your body uses 23 percent of the calories from those foods to process them, storing only 77 percent of every 100 calories eaten. Although excess calories from all food sources are always stored as fat, it is much easier for your body to convert dietary fat into body fat than to turn carbohydrate or protein into body fat.

WHAT IS THE RELATIONSHIP BETWEEN FAT AND ENERGY?

Fat cells do very little work in the body. Their primary function is to store fat, and they perform that task with great efficiency. Normally, your body stores enough fat to sustain you through two or three months of famine conditions. This is fine if you are expecting a famine once or twice a year. The problem with this fat-storage mechanism is that we no longer need it. Of course your body needs a certain amount of fat (for one thing, fatty tissue protects your vital organs).

About 22 percent of a woman's body weight should be from fat; for a man, about 15 percent. If you have more than that, your body must work harder to live. Your heart must pump a greater amount of food and blood through literally miles and miles of blood vessels. Every time you move, your muscles and joints must work harder to carry all the excess baggage. If you don't believe us, try going up a flight of stairs carrying a twenty-five pound bag of potatoes. Then try a fifty-pound bag!

Aside from the well-known health hazards of having too much fat, your energy level is markedly decreased. Your body is too busy working overtime to feed your excess fat cells and to carry around your excess weight to leave you much energy to do anything else.

Do you want more energy? Then get rid of the fat connection.

THE YO-YO SYNDROME

Surely you've wondered why so many people go from diet to diet. Surely you've noticed that the minute people go off a diet they tend to regain the lost weight—and then some—even though they swear they are still eating less. So they try another fad diet, and initially they lose weight again. But history repeats: They gain it all back, along with a few extra pounds.

This process is often called the Yo-Yo Syndrome. Until recently, nutritionists were baffled by it. Their first reaction was to accuse the dieter of "cheating." Ironically, researchers have since discovered what beleaguered dieters knew all along—the dieters were gaining weight even though they were eating less.

WHY DIETS DON'T WORK

Diet researchers originally followed a principle of physics known as the Law of Conservation of Energy. This says that if each day you eat the same number of calories you burn up, your weight will stabilize. According to this principle, to lose weight you simply eat fewer calories than you use. It sounds logical, but it doesn't work. The reason lies with a fascinating mechanism called the set point, which operates something like the thermostat on your home heating system. Instead of setting a temperature level, however, it sets a weight level. Its purpose is to speed or slow your metabolism—to adjust your body's "fuel" system to the amount of food that is available. Thus the thermostat of the set point keeps your weight hovering around a specific level. That level is set genetically. But you can reset it by following the appropriate lifestyle.

The set point was a life-saving mechanism during mankind's hunter-gatherer days, when periods of famine were not uncommon. When the number of calories eaten is reduced by approximately 500 a day, the set point automatically slows down your metabolism. This means that the body is able to burn fewer calories to get the same amount of energy, and store the excess as fat. This helped early man survive times of food scarcity. Unfortunately, the set point mechanism doesn't realize that for most people the days of life-threatening famine are over. So when you start to diet and cut your food intake by, say, 500 calories a day, the set point kicks in, lowers your metabolism, and stores as fat what it sees as excess calories. Depressingly, this metabolic rate shift begins within 48 hours after one starts a deprivation diet.

Another depressing factor in weight control is that after you reach the age of twenty, your metabolic rate will slow down about 1 percent a year. Presuming you were at a perfect weight in your teens, if you maintain the same rate of activity and don't eat any more now than you ate then, you will still gain weight because your metabolism is slowing. Anyone over thirty knows what we're talking about. Because a reduced metabolic rate is inevitable, does it mean you should say, "Why fight it? Please pass the ice cream and cookies"? Of course not! For there is something you can do to counteract it.

EXERCISE RESETS YOUR SET POINT

Even though your set point is originally determined by your genetic inheritance, you can adjust it by your lifestyle. Cardiovascular exercise five times a week will reset your set point so that it "recognizes" a lower weight as your "normal" weight and does not trigger lowered metabolism. Exercise also provides an immediate *increase* in your metabolic rate, and the beneficial fat-burning effects last for hours.

Note from Dave

I was always thin until I went into the army in my early twenties. Until then I could literally eat thousands of calories and my body would burn off the excess. When I returned home from overseas I was extremely upset to find I could no longer fit into my civilian clothes!

I forgot about that early "weight trauma" until one day not long ago when Joely's brother, who's in his early twenties, came to visit us. The whole family noticed that he appeared to be getting a little heavy. "I never gain weight no matter what I eat," he said. "My body burns off the excess." However, challenged by the family's remarks, he went upstairs and got on the scale. He had gained ten pounds. You should have seen his face. Nature had begun to have her way with his metabolism!

The Never Be Tired Again program is designed to combat this metabolic "aging" by helping you shed excess fat and increase your lean muscle tissue. Muscles, in contrast to fat storage cells, burn calories. Thus the more lean muscle tissue you have, the higher your metabolism and the higher the rate at which your cells use oxygen. Higher oxygen consumption, in turn, means higher production of ATP energy molecules. If at the same time you take in less fat, your body will start to burn the excess fat reserves you have accumulated over the years. But the process is not possible unless you do regular cardiovascular exercises such as those we outline in Part IV.

We know this regimen works because graduates of our program have seen the results. They all lost fat and gained lean muscle. Even those who did not lose much weight during the seven-day measuring period did lose a lot of inches. Muscle tissue weighs more than fat, but it is longer and leaner. So even though the scale didn't show the difference within the short seven-day period, this group actually had lost "fat" weight at the same time they gained "muscle" weight.

We remember Ed, who was disappointed at his weighing-in because he lost only four and a half pounds during the seven days. On the other hand, he was extremely pleased because his cholesterol had gone from 282 to 240 and his triglycerides from 279 to 182. On the last night of the program we always have a dress-up dinner. Ed came to dinner with a big grin on his face. "Take a look at this shirt collar!" he exclaimed as he held it about two inches out from his neck. "I just bought a dozen custom-made shirts this size . . . best money I ever wasted!" Then he showed us the waist of his trousers. "I feel like I'm wearing someone else's clothes," he chortled. "I had to pull my belt in two notches to keep these pants up. Incredible!" It's not really incredible. It's the synergistic effect of high-energy nutrition and exercise. You can experience these effects too.

The concept of the set-point and the combination of diet and exercise is so important that we repeat it in chapter 18, where we talk about aerobic exercise. It bears repetition. You cannot hear too often that you must combine nutrition and exercise if you want to make lasting changes in your body.

THE FAT/CHOLESTEROL CONNECTION

Cholesterol and fat go together. If you follow the first rule of high-energy nutrition by keeping the fat content of your diet to 20 percent of total caloric intake, you don't need to worry about your cholesterol. You are automatically cutting the amount of cholesterol in your diet. But it is also important to follow the second rule of high-energy nutrition and hold the animal protein content of your diet to no more than 10 percent of your calories. (We discuss dietary protein in detail in chapter 9.) Together, the guidelines limiting animal protein to 10 percent and fat to 20 percent guarantee that you will not have an excessive amount of cholesterol in your diet. You will actually change your body chemistry.

Do you know what your cholesterol count is? You should. You should know the numbers for your blood pressure, cholesterol, triglycerides, and fasting blood sugar level. They are among the most readily available and easiest-to-interpret indices of your health. Almost every major disease will first manifest itself by a rise in one or more of these numbers; if you keep these figures low, your health will be correspondingly high. Many companies now provide these blood tests for their employees. If your employer does not, then have the tests done by your own physician. All he or she needs is a small blood sample; the results are usually ready in twenty-four hours or less.

Ask your doctor for the actual *numbers*. Don't rely on statistical tables that claim, for example, that a cholesterol range of 180 to 300 is "average." True, those are "average" scores. But remember that 45 percent of the average population gets heart disease! Do you really want to be among the "average" in this case? We don't. Especially since the most recent findings have sharply reduced the "averages" for the "healthy" levels.

A new nationwide study reported in the *Journal of the American Medical Association* says the risk of dying from heart disease is definitely linked to even moderately elevated cholesterol levels. Here's a summary of the study's findings:

Cholesterol Level	Death Rate
182–202	29% higher than those with a cholesterol level below 182
203–220	73% higher
221–244	121% higher
245 and above	242% higher

Dr. Jeremiah Stamler of Northwestern University, coauthor of the study, also says the risk of death from heart disease begins at a much earlier age and at much lower cholesterol levels than medical science previously thought. Take a hard look at the following figures and see where you want to be in terms of your cholesterol level.

Cholesterol Level	Disease Status
200 or higher	Atherosclerosis increasing and arteries becoming more and more blocked
160–199	Process of artery blockage has probably stopped but damage remains along with accompanying risk
Below 160	Good chance to reverse the process

WHERE DOES THE FAT IN YOUR DIET COME FROM?

Five food categories are exceptionally high in fat: red meat, dairy products, oils, nuts, and dressings. Here is a quick-reference list for these foods, along with the percentage of their calories that come from fat:

SUMMARY OF THE FAT CONTENT OF COMMON FOODS

Food	Percent of Calories from Fat

FOOD FROM ANIMAL SOURCES

Meat

	Percent of Calories from Fat
Beef	71–81
Exceptions:	
Flank steak, choice grade	33
Hamburger, lean	50
Lamb	66–79
Pork, including bacon and ham	70–78
Exception:	
Canadian bacon, unheated	60
Chicken and turkey	
Light meat, without skin	18–20
Dark meat, without skin	32–37
Duck without skin	55–65
Squab (light meat) without skin	30
Sausage-type meats, including bologna, frankfurters, salami	74–81
Veal	49–61

Eggs and Dairy Products

	Percent of Calories from Fat
Eggs	
White	trace
Yolk	79
Whole egg, poached	64
Butter	99
Cheese: blue, roquefort, cheddar, Parmesan, Swiss	60–75
Exceptions:	
Cream cheese	89
Cottage cheese (4% fat)	35
Cottage cheese (2% fat)	20
Milk	
Buttermilk, cultured	20
Whole milk (3.5% milkfat)	47
Lowfat (2% milkfat)	30
Nonfat or skim (.1% milkfat)	2
Cream, half and half, table cream, heavy whipping cream	78–95
Sour cream, cultured	86
Cream substitutes, nondairy creamers, whipped toppings	50–69
Ice cream	
Store brands	44
Gourmet brands	65

FOOD FROM PLANT SOURCES

Margarine	99
Oils	100
Nuts, seeds	71–87
Exception:	
Chestnuts	6
Oily fruits or vegetables	
Avocados	82
Olives	90

COMBINATION FOODS

Dressings: Blue cheese, French, Russian, Thousand Island	83–97
Sauces: Mayonnaise, tartar sauce	96–98

THIS IS YOUR LIFE: A TWO-ACT PLAY

Let's examine some probably typical experiences in your life that will show how your eating habits provide obvious—and not so obvious—sources of fat:

ACT I: THAT SPECIAL DINNER

You've heard about this great restaurant. It promises to serve you the biggest and best cut of prime rib you've ever had, along with a baked potato swimming in butter and sour cream (or potatoes au gratin), vegetables in a delicious cheese sauce, and cheesy garlic bread. As an appetizer, you'll get the best New England–style clam chowder, and for dessert, something so sinfully rich you'll want seconds no matter how full you are. You think, "Gee, I really have to try that place." Eventually you do.

Haven't you had meals like this? Of course you have. But chances are you never bothered to analyze such a dinner for its fat content. Let's start with the butter, an obvious source of almost 100 percent fat. The sour cream is 86 percent fat. The cheese: approximately 60 to 70 percent fat. That tasty New England chowder is made primarily of medium cream (83 percent fat) and butter.

You were probably taught that prime ribs are a great source of protein, right? Wrong. They're a great source of fat. Eighty-one percent of the calories in a prime rib comes from fat. Protein accounts for only 19 percent of the calories. And when we say 81 percent of the calories come from fat, we don't mean the visible fat around the edge of the meat. We mean the fat that is marbled *into* the meat itself.

And what about the dessert? Even though the restaurant claims you will want two desserts, you feel pretty full from your cheesy garlic bread, soup, and "king's cut" prime rib with potato and vegetables. So instead of ordering the seven-layer chocolate mousse cake with ice cream, you order a "simple" dish of ice cream with fruit. The fruit is healthful enough, but the ice cream is approximately 60 percent fat. All told, between 70 and 80 percent of the calories in your entire meal comes from fat!

Okay, so you don't do that sort of thing very often (or do you?). Then let's take a look at a much less festive occasion.

ACT II: A "DIET" LUNCH

It has been a bad day at the office, and you'll be lucky if you get to eat lunch at your desk. Finally, your stomach is rumbling so loudly you have no choice but to send out for lunch. You're trying to be really careful about your diet, so you order a tuna salad sandwich. You tell them to hold the potato chips and give you coleslaw instead. You resist ordering the ice cream smoothie and settle for a light coffee. But if you analyze your "diet" lunch it turns out to be far from a diet lunch after all. About 60 to 70 percent of your calories are fat, thanks to all the mayonnaise in the tuna salad and coleslaw, and the cream in your coffee.

You can learn to order correctly when eating away from home. You can learn to buy foods that have a low fat content by consulting the list of high-energy foods in chapter 13 and by learning how to read food labels. Packaged and canned foods are required by law to have a nutritional label if anything is added to the food or if the manufacturer makes any nutritional claims for it. (It is ironic that while not all food for human consumption is legally required to have a nutritional label, pet foods are legally required to list all ingredients and provide an analysis of the contents!)

TEN THINGS YOU NEED TO KNOW ABOUT SQUEEZING THE FAT OUT OF YOUR DIET

1. HOW TO CALCULATE FAT CONTENT FROM A LABEL

Determining the fat content of packaged or canned foods is simple if you can handle a little math (or have a calculator). Remember these basic facts:

1 gram fat = 9 calories
1 gram carbohydrate = 4 calories
1 gram protein = 4 calories

For practice, follow the step-by-step example below and then try analyzing some of the food labels in your kitchen cabinets.

Low-fat Milk (2% Milkfat)
Nutrition Information Per Serving

Serving Size	one cup
Servings Per Container	4
Calories	140
Protein	10 GRAMS
Carbohydrate	13 GRAMS
Fat	5 GRAMS
Sodium	150 mg

Ingredients: MILK, SKIM, NONFAT MILK SOLIDS, VITAMIN A PALMITATE AND VITAMIN D_3

---

1. Note the calories per serving listed on the label. In the example of low-fat milk shown above there are 140 calories per serving.
2. Multiply the grams of fat in each serving by 9. This gives you the number of calories per serving that come from fat. In this example 45 calories in each serving come from fat (5 grams of fat multiplied by 9 calories per gram).
3. Divide the fat calories by the calories per serving. (This is where a calculator comes in handy, unless you remember your long division.) In this example, 45 calories of fat divided by 140 calories per serving equals .32, or 32 percent. This is far too much to meet the high-energy standard maximum of 20 percent fat.

Now look at the low-fat milk label again. Notice the phrase "2% Milkfat." Are you a little confused? If the label says 2 percent, how come our calculations show that low-fat milk is actually 32 percent fat? The answer lies in a definition of terms. The milk producer is being honest but defines fat as a percentage of volume or weight. We are talking about fat as a percentage of calories. Most of the volume of low-fat milk consists of water; therefore fat considered as volume accounts for only 2 percent of the total volume. But when you consider calories—which we contend is a more realistic and healthier standard to use—the calories in low-fat milk that are attributable to fat make up more than 30 percent of the total calories. This makes all the difference in the world when you're trying to manage the percentage of fat in your diet!

Meat producers are also trying to portray their products in the best possible light by labeling ground meat like hamburger as "extra lean ground beef, does not exceed 15 percent fat." Don't be deceived. They, too, are referring to fat as a percentage of weight. In one of our local supermarkets you can find a package of ground turkey labeled "93 percent fat free" in large letters, and with "7 percent fat" in much smaller type. If you examine the nutritional label on the back, you will discover that of the 140 calories per serving, there are 7 grams of fat. This means that 45 percent of the calories in the turkey come from fat. (Seven grams of fat times 9 calories per gram equals 63. Divide 63 by 140 calories per serving to get 45 percent.) A little bit different from 7 percent!

Miracles Never Cease
Notes from Joely

I was shocked when I learned that all those wonderful dairy products I had substituted for red meat in my diet had just as much fat and cholesterol as meat. In a moment of unrestrained fervor I vowed to switch to nonfat milk for my morning cereal. My fervor was dampened considerably when I poured my first serving of nonfat milk. Good grief, it was gray! Even worse, it tasted gray! Nevertheless I resolved to be stalwart. I put gray milk on my cereal every morning for a week, and every morning for a week I was angry when I sat down to breakfast.

I finally decided that discretion was the better part of valor. I switched to 2 percent milk, which at 32 percent fat had a much higher fat content than I wanted but was still better than the 50 percent fat of whole milk. What's more, it looked and tasted like milk. I lived very happily with the 2 percent milk for a couple of months until the day I arrived at the grocery store prior to the delivery of the 2 percent milk. Should I be a good girl and take the nonfat milk, or should I listen to my taste buds, grab the whole milk, and run?

My decision was fairly easy, not because I'm such a good person but because I knew David would be reading the labels. So I bought the nonfat milk. Miracles never cease. When I tried it the next morning, it wasn't so bad. They obviously had changed the formula, I told myself. It couldn't possibly be, could it, that my tastes had changed with the gradual withdrawal of fat content?

It is my experience that many people react to diet changes much the same way. If after you make an effort to lower the fat content of your milk you feel that life is not worth living without whole milk on your cereal, then *don't* change (at least not just yet). Make diet changes you can live with at first, and gradually work up to the others. You know the areas in your life where you can make "cold turkey" changes. Do that, and then be gentle with yourself, moving gradually where the "sacred diet cows" in your life are concerned.

2. FROZEN DIET DINNERS ARE OFTEN HIGH IN FAT

Let's examine one more packaged food label. If you were asked whether a frozen diet dinner was low in fat, what would you say? Most people look at the number of calories on the label and decide that low calories mean low fat.

But look at the labels and decide for yourself. A diet oven-fried fish dinner with vegetables has 220 calories per serving. But of its 220 calories, 108 are fat, or 49 percent of the calorie count. A diet southern fried chicken patty dinner has 270 calories. Someone who is counting calories might not think to look at the fat content, but it weighs in at 18 grams, or 60 percent of the 270 calories in the patty. Another example is a diet beef and pork frozen dinner with sauce, which is 33 percent fat! Microwave breaded cod lists 290 calories per serving in bold letters on the package. You must read the label carefully to notice that the package contains two servings. Whether you eat one or two servings, however, you are eating 19 grams of fat per serving, which means 59 percent of your calories are from fat.

3. PREPARATION OF GOOD NUTRITION NEEDN'T BE TIME-CONSUMING

There is help for the weary. If you are exhausted at the end of your working day and consider frozen "diet" dinners an absolute lifesaver, you are probably alternating between despair and anger as you read this. What, exactly, do we expect you to eat?

Fortunately, good nutrition can be easy to prepare. Here's an example: Put fish in a covered dish with one-eighth to one-quarter inch of white wine or nonfat milk. If you like wine, the alcohol cooks off and you're left with a wonderful taste. If you can't stand the odor of cooking fish, choose the milk option: Milk absorbs the odor and keeps the fish moist at the same time. Regardless of which liquid you choose, bake the fish at 425 degrees for eight to twelve minutes, depending on the thickness of the fish. (Frozen dinners take longer than that to cook.) Put some potatoes in the microwave and serve with "healthy sour cream" (see recipe #37), parsley, chives, a little low-salt salsa, some Dijon mustard if you're a mustard fan (even a touch of mustard can be tasty if you're not a big fan), some meatless chili, grated raw zucchini, summer squash, beets, carrots . . . The list is almost endless. More important, this dinner doesn't take hours and a culinary-school degree to prepare.

4. THERE ARE GOOD LOW-FAT ALTERNATIVES TO DAIRY PRODUCTS

Fortunately, the dairy industry has already come up with low-fat and nonfat versions of milk, yogurt, and cottage cheese. The difference between low-fat and nonfat versions can be confusing, so read the labels. In order to stay at 20 percent fat or lower, buy nonfat or skim milk that has approximately 2 percent of its calories in fat. Look for milk that is labeled ".1 percent fat." It will be less than 20 percent fat by calories. Lowfat cottage cheese and nonfat yogurt are both 20 percent fat.

You can make a quite acceptable substitute for sour cream using low-fat cottage cheese and/or nonfat yogurt. Whip the low-fat cottage cheese in the blender. If you like your "sour cream" a little tart, add plain nonfat yogurt. Finish with a dash of lemon juice. You can also add garlic powder or mustard for more flavor. Our favorite version uses Gourmet Sprinkle as a flavor enhancer. (See the shopping list in chapter 23 for further information.) This makes a wonderful dip for vegetables and is a big hit at parties.

Both butter and margarine are 100 percent fat and have about the same number of calories. The difference between them is that margarine comes from vegetable sources and therefore has no cholesterol. Again, however, you must read the label. *Many margarines are made with hydrogenated oil, which causes the body to produce cholesterol.* So even though these margarines don't *contain* cholesterol, the hydrogenation process saturates the oil, and saturated fat causes the body to manufacture cholesterol. In place of butter or margarine on your toast or muffin, try some of the jams that are made out of fruit only, with no added sugar or sweeteners. There are several delicious brands available. Health food stores will have the widest selection, but supermarkets are catching on, too.

There are no real alternatives to cheese if you like your cheese in the form of crackers and cheese and cheese sauces. Cheese has as much fat as red meat. Even "reduced fat" cheese—the kind that promises to save you 50 percent of the calories of regular cheese— gets a whopping 40 percent of its calories from fat. If you are willing to cut down on the amount of cheese, sprinkling a little parmesan on your pasta or vegetables will give you a nice taste and still be within the 20 percent fat limit.

5. HUMPTY DUMPTY EGGS CAN SAVE YOU A LOT OF FAT

Separate your egg whites and yolks. Don't let the king's men put them together again. You've just saved yourself 79 percent fat. The egg yolk is 79 percent fat, while the white of the egg is virtually fat-free. You can improve the fat content of any recipe that calls for eggs by eliminating the yolk and doubling the number of egg whites. For example, if a recipe calls for two eggs, use four egg whites.

Are you wondering what to do with the yolks? In every seminar we have ever given, someone asks that question. The answer is, "Throw them away." A dozen eggs cost somewhere in the vicinity of $1.20. By throwing out the yolk, you are "throwing out" 60 cents—and possibly saving yourself thousands of dollars in future medical bills. If you really can't stand throwing out all the yolks, give an occasional yolk to your dog or cat—it will help your pet maintain a healthy coat.

6. ONE MAN'S MEAT TRULY IS ANOTHER MAN'S POISON

Red meat is a major source of dietary fat. The white meat of chicken, on the other hand, has less than 20 percent fat if you don't eat the skin. Turkey is another white meat that has less than 20 percent fat. Fish, of course, is an excellent alternative to meat; white fish and shellfish have less than 20 percent fat. Darker fish like mackerel, Atlantic herring, Norwegian sardines, rainbow trout, swordfish, and salmon have a higher percentage of fat, but it's a beneficial kind of fat. These fish have large amounts of omega-3 fatty acids, a substance that has been shown to increase HDL (good cholesterol) and decrease LDL (bad cholesterol). Scientists discovered the beneficial effects of omega-3 fatty acids while studying Eskimos, who live on a diet extremely high in fat yet have virtually none of the cardiovascular problems associated with high-fat diets. This seemed to fly in the face of what science knew about fat, cholesterol, and heart disease until the researchers discovered that omega-3 fatty acids appeared to provide a magic shield against those diseases.

You probably have been told that you shouldn't eat shellfish because it is high in cholesterol. We now know that early research erred by lumping fish sterols and cholesterol together. Fish sterols do not clog arteries the way cholesterol does. So don't worry about shellfish: It is low in cholesterol and low in fat (as long as you don't drown it in butter, bread it and fry it, or smother it in mayonnaise-saturated tartar sauce).

According to William S. Harris, a nutritional researcher at the University of Oregon, fish oils have been found to:

- Lower cholesterol
- Lower triglycerides, which are fatty acids in the bloodstream
- Help relieve inflammatory conditions such as eczema, psoriasis, and arthritis
- Lower blood pressure
- Help prevent blood clots

7. THERE IS A LOW-FAT WAY TO FRY

Even if you've given up deep frying your food (which we certainly hope you have), you may still sauté in butter or oil on the theory that you're getting a lot less fat. You can reduce the amount of fat even more, and still get great flavor, by sautéing in defatted chicken broth or vegetable broth. Simply spray the frying pan with Pam or Mazola Spray Oil. Then brown the food very quickly and add a small amount of broth. You can sauté onions, peppers, mushrooms, etc. this way quite easily. They taste delicious and are virtually fat-free.

8. THERE ARE GOOD SUBSTITUTES FOR OIL IN RECIPES

Most recipes for baked goods call for oil and sugar. You can avoid using both if you substitute for the oil the same amount of a fruit concentrate. Then you don't have to add sugar at all. For example, if a recipe calls for two tablespoons of oil and one tablespoon of sugar, add two tablespoons of apple concentrate and no sugar. Your taste buds will never know the difference, but your body will. Fruit concentrate is available in most health food stores. There are several brands and they all come in bottles. Flavors include apple, grape, blackberry, and cranberry. Because they are fruit concentrates they react differently in your body from sugar. (We'll talk more about sugar in chapter 12.)

9. YOU MUST BE SELECTIVE ABOUT SALAD DRESSINGS

How often have you ordered a salad for lunch because you're on another one of your perennial diets? You go to the salad bar and pile your plate with raw veggies. So far, so good. Then you get to the salad dressings and put two big scoops of blue cheese, creamy Italian, or Thousand Island dressing on the salad. You have just succeeded in turning a meal that was 5 to 10 percent fat into one that is about 85 percent fat!

Before you buy reduced-calorie salad dressings, read their labels. You'll find many of them are still high in fat. Take a look at the salad dressings in chapter 23 for some ideas on how you can make your own low-fat dressings.

10. YOU MUST CHECK THE LABELS WHEN YOU BUY SNACKS

Supermarket-purchased snacks are usually high in fat *and* high in sugar. Even if they say "no cholesterol," in all likelihood they contain hydrogenated oils, which, as we mentioned earlier, stimulate your body to produce cholesterol. On the other hand, you can find healthful snack foods in health food stores if you read your labels carefully. But don't let the phrase "health food store" lull you into complacency. Health food stores also carry a lot of "fatty" snack foods with healthy-sounding descriptions like "wheat-free" or "organic." See chapter 23 for a list of high-energy foods to snack on. Also, pay attention to the list of low-energy foods in chapter 12. Avoid them like the plague!

Chapter 9

Protein and Energy: New Answers to Some Old Misconceptions

Here's a quick quiz to test your knowledge of protein.

1. Protein is found only in meat, fish, eggs, and dairy products.   True False

2. The major nutritional component of meat is protein.   True False

3. The major nutritional component of dairy products is protein.   True False

4. High cholesterol always goes with high fat content.   True False

5. If you want to lose weight, it's a good idea to eat the hamburger and leave the bun.   True False

The correct answer to each of these statements is . . . *False*. That's right, every single one is false. Clearly, protein is one of the most misunderstood subjects in nutrition. Let's examine the statements above in detail and see if we can't clear up some of those mistaken impressions.

WHERE DOES PROTEIN COME FROM? HOW MUCH DO YOU NEED?

Most people will say protein comes from meat. If they are a bit better informed, they may tell you protein also comes from fish, eggs, and dairy products. Not too many folks will say that protein also is found in vegetables, fruits, grains, beans, and nuts. Take a look at the amazing amount of protein in the foods listed below. (All of the numbers derive from extensive research by the U.S. Department of Agriculture.)

Food— 100 grams (3.5 oz.)	% Protein	Grams Protein	% Fat	% Carbohydrate*
Almonds	11	18.6	76	13
Broccoli, raw	27	3.6	8	66
Grapes, Concord	6	1.3	12	82
Green peas, cooked	26	2.9	5	69
Lentils, split	25	24.7	2	74
Mushrooms	25	2.7	9	55
Oatmeal	13	2.0	15	73
Pinto beans (dry)	26	22.9	3	72
Potatoes, baked in skin	8	2.6	1	91
Snap green beans	16	1.6	8	76
Zucchini	29	1.2	13	57

*Combined percentages of protein, fat, and carbohydrate may not all add up to 100 percent because of rounding off of figures.

According to the National Academy of Sciences—National Research Council, you need much less protein than you are probably getting now. Males between the ages of eleven and fourteen need 45 grams of protein a day. From fifteen on, males need 56 grams a day. This is only two ounces. Females between eleven and eighteen need 46 grams of protein a day. From nineteen on, the protein requirement for females actually drops to 44 grams a day, which amounts to one and a half ounces.

Though we need only relatively small amounts of it, protein is vital to the human body. It is used to repair cells and promote the growth of new cells. Protein is manufactured in the body from amino acids. Your body can make all of the amino acids from carbohydrates and nitrogen, except for nine so-called "essential" amino acids. They're called "essential" because they must come from protein in the food we eat. Although meat contains the greatest number of essential amino acids, you don't have to eat meat to get them. Vegetables also contain the essential amino acids.

Another major misconception about protein has to do with "complete" and "incomplete" protein. Animal protein is said to be "complete" because it contains a balance of all nine amino acids. Vegetable protein is supposedly "incomplete" because its amino acids are not in the same balance as in animal protein. Some vegetables contain more of one essential amino acid while other vegetables contain more of another. But new nutritional research has discovered that your body doesn't need all nine amino acids at once. Your body can store them in an amino acid "pool" in the liver and withdraw the amino acids it needs to manufacture protein.

Thus, as long as your body gets all nine essential amino acids, the source doesn't matter. All food is broken down into chemical molecules during digestion. It doesn't matter whether the essential amino acids come from animal sources or plant sources. Your body treats them the same way and uses them in the same way.

MEAT IS *NOT* A GOOD SOURCE OF PROTEIN

If it doesn't matter where we get the nine essential amino acids, what's all the fuss about meat? The truth is that meat (especially red meat) and dairy products are not particularly efficient sources of protein. They are great sources of fat. And you definitely want to avoid large quantities of fat. Here is a breakdown of the protein and fat content of some meat and dairy products.

PROTEIN VS. FAT CONTENT OF COMMON MEATS AND DAIRY PRODUCTS

	% Protein	Grams Protein	% Fat
Meat 100 grams (3.5 oz.)— less than ¼ pound			
Bacon, broiled or fried and drained	20	30.4	77
T-bone, Choice grade, broiled	16	19.5	82
Bologna, all meat	19	13.3	74
Frankfurters, all meat	18	13.1	78
Ham, thin class, roasted	28	24.2	70
Pork loin, fat class, roasted	24	23.5	74
Pork spareribs, medium fat class	16	14.5	83

Dairy Products
100 grams (3.5 oz.)—
less than ½ cup

Whole milk (3.5% Milkfat)	22	3.5	48
Skim (nonfat)	40	3.6	2
American cheese, processed	25	23.2	73
Blue, roquefort types	23	21.5	73
Egg, whole	32	12.9	64
Egg white	93	10.9	trace

It's obvious from these figures that meat and dairy products are much better sources of fat than of protein. Does this mean you should never eat red meat or dairy products again? Of course not. It does mean that you should limit the amount you eat. There are excellent sources of protein that do not carry the same fat penalty that meat does. You can get the calcium that dairy products provide from nonfat dairy products, from other foods, and from supplements without all the fat that goes with whole milk products.

In addition to its high fat content, meat contains other ingredients that are equally unappetizing. According to *The New England Journal of Medicine,* 40 percent of the antibiotics produced in this country for the last thirty years have been fed to animals. The

PROTEIN VS. FAT CONTENT OF SELECTED SEAFOODS

	% Protein	Grams Protein	% Fat
Fish, Shellfish 100 grams (3.5 oz.), raw			
Catfish	68	17.6	27
Cod	90	17.6	10
Crab, blue Dungeness, rock, king, steamed	74	17.3	18
Flounder, sole	85	16.7	9
Haddock	93	18.3	1
Lobster, northern	74	17.3	19
Mackerel	40	19.0	57
Salmon, pink	67	20.0	28
Oysters, eastern	51	8.4	25

routine use of penicillin and tetracycline in animal feed is creating a serious medical problem because the infectious microbes that prevail in the community are developing an immunity to the drugs. Thus, when you or your child need antibiotics to kill an invading virus, they may not be as effective as they should be. Consequently, doctors often find it necessary to use higher dosages of antibiotics in medical treatments. The fact is that we just don't know the long-term risks of routinely consuming meat containing hidden antibiotics.

Fish, on the other hand, is an excellent source of protein and, for the most part, is extremely low in fat.

A POSTSCRIPT ON CHOLESTEROL

We've been talking about where protein comes from. Do you know where cholesterol comes from? It occurs in any food of animal origin: all meat, fish, eggs, and dairy products. Anything that can walk, crawl, swim, or fly has cholesterol. Conversely, anything that comes from plants has no cholesterol. There is never any cholesterol in vegetables, fruits, grains, nuts, beans, or any oil made from these foods. Even when a food is 100 percent fat, like olive oil or safflower oil, it contains no cholesterol. That's a major reason why total vegetarians have extremely low cholesterol.

THREE FACTS ABOUT EATING TOO MUCH PROTEIN

1. TOO MUCH PROTEIN CAN MAKE YOU TIRED

What happens when you fill a glass too full of water? The excess gets wasted. The same is true of protein. To begin with, your body doesn't store protein as such; rather, it breaks down protein into its amino acids and stores them in the amino acid pool. Even so, the body can store only a limited amount of amino acids. When you don't need any more protein to repair the body and to build new cells, nitrogen is removed from the protein molecule and converted into uric acid. Since uric acid is a poison, the body excretes it in urine. After the nitrogen—which is what makes a protein molecule different from other molecules—has been removed, the molecule is no longer protein. Therefore the body treats it like any other energy source: It considers it merely as excess calories. These are then stored where all other excess calories go—on your hips, thighs, and waistline in the familiar form of fat.

To top it off, your body draws water from the cells to help flush the uric acid out of your system. This, in turn, upsets the magnesium-potassium balance in your cells and can cause tiredness. Flushing the uric acid out of your body also puts a strain on your kidneys. Chronic kidney strain can lead to serious medical problems later in life.

2. TOO MUCH PROTEIN CAN LEAD TO CALCIUM LOSS

Do you remember all those television commercials that talked about the importance of the "pH balance" in your shampoo? Well, the pH balance—the proportion of acids and alkalines—of your blood is far more important. Excess protein makes your blood more acidic. To help balance the blood's acid/alkaline level, your bones give up some of their calcium. But your bones need that calcium to keep them strong, and the loss of calcium increases the risk of osteoporosis. That's another reason why people who eat the hamburger and leave the bun as part of their attempt to diet are doing themselves a disservice. First of all, the fat content of the hamburger is somewhere around 50 percent, as opposed to the bread's fat content, which is under 20 percent. Second, burger eaters are more than likely adding excess protein to their already overburdened systems.

3. TOO MUCH PROTEIN INCREASES YOUR RISK OF CANCER

The third item of bad news about excess protein has to do with cancer. No doubt you are sick and tired of hearing that everything causes cancer. However, isn't it better to be sick and tired of hearing about cancer and be able to do something to prevent it, than to be sick and tired because you have it? With protein, it's only the excess that needs to concern you. Some experts claim you can't separate the cancer-causing effects of fat and protein, since most sources of protein in fact have greater amounts of fat than protein. But laboratory tests that can separate fat from protein indicate that animal protein promotes cancer even more dramatically than fat does. To be on the safe side, limit the animal sources of protein in your diet. Here's an easy way to figure out how much that is.

A SIMPLE RULE OF THUMB

We should probably call this a "rule of fist," because that's how you determine how much meat or fish you should eat. Make a fist and look at the top of your hand from the edge of the wrist to the knuckles. That's how much fish or meat you should have in a day. (If your friend gets a bigger piece than you do because he or she has a bigger fist, you have to realize that your friend is probably bigger than you to begin with. So a little more protein is appropriate.) Also, the piece of fish or meat should be no more than half an inch thick.

If you're used to eating meat two or three times a day, you're probably wondering, "What the heck am I going to eat instead?" The menus for the seven-day program in chapter 10 will give you ideas for alternatives. It really is a matter of attitude. Be open to the possibility that you will find healthy alternatives you will enjoy eating as much, if not more than, your usual choices.

GOOD NEWS: NO MORE SLEEPY AFTERNOONS!

We've all been there: the big business lunch meeting followed by an afternoon of trying to stay awake to meet that last-minute deadline! There are two main reasons for this scenario. First, you may have eaten too large and too fatty a meal. This results in your brain's being deprived of an adequate blood supply because all your energy is now focused on digesting that meal. Second, your tiredness may be due to the fact that you ate a lot of carbohydrates in the form of breads, sugary desserts, and alcohol. Judith Wurtman, Ph.D., of MIT, has found that a meal high in carbohydrates can slow you down. This is particularly true for women.

The way to avoid these problems is simple:

- Eat a fairly light lunch that derives not more than 10 percent of its calories from animal protein and at least 65 to 70 percent from vegetables.

- Eat at least some of the protein first. If you eat carbohydrates first, you get sleepy.
- Make sure your lunch does not have more than 20 percent of its calories from fat.
- Skip breads, sugary deserts, and alcohol.

Then watch your afternoon energy level zoom!

QUICK ENERGY CHARGE #4

A High-Energy Lunch

Steps 1–5: See the instructions preceding Quick Energy Charge #1 in chapter 4.

Step 6: Energy Programming

Breathing slowly and deeply, see the oxygen entering every cell in your body. See your tiredness and tension melting into the grass, leaving you relaxed and alert. With each breath, breathe in increased energy and breathe out tiredness and stress. See the energy come into your body as pure white light.

Now that your deepest self is tuned in and harmonizing in this relaxed but alert state, imagine yourself going into your favorite business luncheon restaurant. Sense that you are feeling good about the meeting and know that after it is concluded you will go back to the office refreshed and rejuvenated. See yourself ordering your favorite fish, broiled with garlic (no oil, no butter); your favorite vegetable lightly steamed without oil or butter; and a salad with vinegar and olive oil dressing served on the side. Actually taste the gourmet flavor of this, your favorite high-energy business lunch. Delicious!

See yourself leave the meeting and return to your office feeling light and energetic. Imagine watching yourself as you exhibit incredible stamina and productivity, getting incredible energy as your body digests your lunch cleanly and efficiently. Feel the warmth and intense satisfaction from knowing you have mastered the art of power lunching!

Step 7: Reentry. See the instructions preceding Quick Energy Charge #1 in chapter 4.

Chapter 10

The Seven-Day Energy-Building Program

Can you recall when you last set aside some special time in which to pay full attention to yourself and your own needs? If you are like most people, you're going to say, "I can't remember *when* I had a chance to do that. The demands of my job and my family just don't allow me that luxury."

We submit that devoting quality time to taking care of your personal well-being is not a luxury, but a necessity. In the long run, the results will make you a more energetic and productive worker and a happier and more loving partner and parent.

Our proven seven-day energy-building program is your opportunity to give yourself permission to center all of your attention on yourself, even if only for a week. Ideally, to fulfill the program's goals most effectively, you should take the seven days away from work (or your other normal weekly routines). If that is not possible, you can still follow the program at a less intensive level.

Carrying out any part of the program is better than doing nothing. One step forward puts you one step farther ahead than you were before you took that step. So don't be discouraged if you need to take more than seven days to carry out the program. To enable you to fit the program into your schedule, we have organized it into three levels of intensity. Remember, the seven-day energy-building program is meant to serve as a launching pad for your permanent lifestyle change. It is a beginning, not an end. If you can take a week away from your normal schedule, you can expect to see dramatic results in terms of weight change and measurement changes; decreases in cholesterol, triglyceride, and blood pressure readings; and increases in your energy level. If you need to begin your change more gradually, you can still expect to get the same results—but in proportion to the time you are able to take to make these changes. It will be the best investment you ever made!

GETTING READY TO BOOST YOUR ENERGY

Before you begin the seven-day program, there are several important preparatory steps you need to take.

1. *Get a medical checkup* to find out your cholesterol, triglyceride, and blood sugar levels. Your physician will probably want to make this a "fasting" blood test, so make an early morning appointment. These readings, along with your blood pressure numbers, provide the baseline data you need to see the dramatic changes that will take place during the seven-day program. Then make a second appointment for a follow-up blood test after you have done the basic program.

2. *Make sure your physician approves* of your participation in the exercise component of the program. Ask about potassium supplements if you feel you will be perspiring more than normal, since increased fluid loss can upset your potassium balance and cause tiredness.

3. *Know what your energy-building heart rate is* (read chapter 19 to find out how to ascertain this). Learn how to take your pulse before, during, and after each exercise session. You will not get the benefits of cardiovascular exercise if your heart rate is not what it should be. If you have difficulty taking your pulse accurately, consider buying a pulse meter. Several kinds are available: One attaches to a bicycle exerciser or treadmill and costs about $120; another is a watch with a chest strap and costs about $250. More expensive models feed data into your computer and analyze your progress. Whether you choose to take your pulse yourself or buy a pulse meter, it is important to monitor your heart rate if you want to get the full benefit of cardiovascular exercise.

4. *Make sure you have comfortable exercise shoes.* The biggest health concern we find in our live-in program has always been blisters. Few things are as much of a *dis*incentive to exercise as bleeding blisters.

5. *Plan a varied program of exercise.* Levels 2 and 3 of the seven-day energy-building program call for more than one exercise

period a day. Each type of physical activity we recommend in chapter 20—walking, swimming, bicycling—exercises different muscles in different ways. If you select more than one kind of cardiovascular exercise you will give your body a more thorough workout, and save yourself from the sore muscles that may result from doing only one type of exercise. The stretching component of the program will also help keep your muscles from getting stiff.

6. *Plan your food shopping to match the recipes you select.* Don't wait until the last minute to find you don't have the proper ingredients, and end up substituting the wrong alternatives.

7. If you can take a week for yourself, *plan on getting at least one massage,* or preferably several over the course of the week. It's a good idea, too, to soak in a relaxing warm bath or use a whirlpool once a day.

8. *Anticipate adjustments in your digestive system.* On the Never Be Tired Again nutritional program you will probably be getting more fiber in your diet than you usually eat. This may cause some gas and bloating at first, but the condition will pass as your body adjusts to the healthier fiber level. Increased water consumption helps to reduce this temporary affliction. Drink at least eight glasses of water each day. Cool water is absorbed more quickly; carbonated water enters the bloodstream faster than regular water. Try flavored carbonated water rather than diet soft drinks, which contain chemicals and artificial sweeteners.

9. *Ask your doctor or nutritionist to recommend a good multivitamin/ multimineral supplement.* Since most of the people who take our seven-day program want to lose weight, the calorie level is lower for the program than a maintenance diet should be. Therefore, it is important that you take a multivitamin/multimineral supplement. When you finish the seven-day program, increase the amount of food that you eat, but observe the five rules of high-energy nutrition discussed in chapter 7.

HOW TO CHOOSE YOUR STARTING POINT

There are three levels in the seven-day energy-building program. Each is based on two criteria: One is your total score on the High-Energy Lifestyle Inventory (HELI) in chapter 2, and the other is your cholesterol level. Begin your personal program at the highest level at which one of your scores appears. If, for example, your HELI score puts you in Level 2 but your cholesterol reading puts you in Level 3, follow the Level 3 schedule.

Level 1
Total HELI score: 495–560
Cholesterol: less than 160

Level 2
Total HELI score: 326–494
Cholesterol: 160–199

Level 3
Total HELI score: 80–325
Cholesterol: 200 and over

LEVEL 1: SEVEN-DAY SCHEDULE

You can follow Level 1 of the seven-day energy-building program while you go about your normal weekly routine. Although it is preferable to devote this time exclusively to taking care of your well-being, you can continue to go to work and still participate fully at this level. If you do, do the stretches in the evening if you don't have time for them after your morning cardiovascular workout. The schedule for Level One begins on page 110.

LEVEL 2: SEVEN-DAY SCHEDULE

Level 2 of the seven-day energy-building program is moderately intense. Even so, you should plan on taking seven days away from your regular schedule if at all possible in order to participate fully in this program. There are two exercise periods per day. The schedule for Level Two begins on page 117.

LEVEL 3: SEVEN-DAY SCHEDULE

Level 3 is a highly intensive program designed to quickly lower your cholesterol, help you lose weight and inches, decrease feelings of anxiety and stress, and increase your energy. Level 3 includes three exercise periods each day and two quick-energy charges. Because of this program's intensity, you *must* be able to take seven consecutive days away from your normal schedule. The schedule for Level Three begins on page 124.

LEVEL 1: DAY 1

Before breakfast

Energy-building exercise
Choose one: walking—40 minutes
treadmill—30 minutes
swimming—30 minutes
stationary bike—20 minutes
jogging—20 minutes

Breakfast

Hot Cereal with Raisins (recipe #1)
Beverage (see recommended beverages, chapter 23)

**Mid-morning quick
energy charge**

Quick Energy Charge #1 (see chapter 4). Quick energy
charges should not be done on a full stomach; wait
until your previous meal has settled.

Mid-morning snack

Your choice (see recommended snacks, chapter 23)

Lunch

Double Decker Sandwich (recipe #8)
Beverage

**Mid-afternoon quick
energy charge**

Quick Energy Charge #2 (see chapter 6)

Mid-afternoon snack

Raw vegetables, especially carrot strips

Dinner

Poached Salmon with Tomato Caper Sauce (recipe
#21)
Domino Potatoes (recipe #29)
Sweet and Tangy Carrots (recipe #28)
Beverage

Evening snack/dessert

Baked Apple with Raisins (recipe #48)

Stretch for energy

See chapter 21 for stretches

Personal pampering

Every day try one or more of the following suggestions
for personal pampering:
Soak in tub/whirlpool
Sauna/steambath
Manicure/pedicure
Facial
Massage
Get your hair done/new hairstyle

DAILY NUTRITIONAL SCORECARD
Calories: 1363

NUTRIENT	Carbohydrate	Fat	Total Protein	Animal Protein
PERCENT CALORIES	73%	9%	15%	7%
AMOUNT	257.9 G	14.5 G	53.0 G	22.7 G

Note: If you do not want to lose weight or if you are extremely active physically, you may want to
increase the number of calories that you consume each day. You can do this without sacrificing
your opportunity to improve your energy level if you get your additional calories from eating grains,
vegetables, and fruits.

LEVEL 1: DAY 2

Before breakfast	Energy-building exercise
Breakfast	Cold Cereal with Fruit (recipe #2) Beverage
Mid-morning quick energy charge	Quick Energy Charge #3 (see chapter 7)
Mid-morning snack	Snack of your choice (see approved list)
Lunch	Quinoa-Tomato Soup (recipe #11) Luncheon Salad with Pesto (recipe #33) Beverage
Mid-afternoon quick energy charge	Quick Energy Charge #4 (see chapter 9)
Mid-afternoon snack	Raw vegetables, especially carrot strips
Dinner	Chicken with Fettucine (recipe #14) Spinach with Feta Cheese (recipe #26) Beverage
Evening snack/dessert	Two California Orbap Cookies (recipe #45)
Stretch for energy	See chapter 21 for stretches
Personal pampering	Your choice: Soak in tub/whirlpool Sauna/steambath Manicure/pedicure Facial Massage Get your hair done/new hairstyle

DAILY NUTRITIONAL SCORECARD
Carories: 1442

NUTRIENT	Carbohydrate	Fat	Total Protein	Animal Protein
PERCENT CALORIES	70%	10%	19%	9%
AMOUNT	259.2 G	16.5 G	70.8 G	34 G

Note: If you do not want to lose weight or if you are extremely active physically, you may want to increase the number of calories that you consume each day. You can do this without sacrificing your opportunity to improve your energy level if you get your additional calories from eating grains, vegetables, and fruits.

LEVEL 1: DAY 3

Before breakfast	Energy-building exercise
Breakfast	Hot Cereal with Raisins (recipe #1) Beverage
Mid-morning quick energy charge	Quick Energy Charge #5 (see chapter 12)
Mid-morning snack	Snack of your choice (see approved list)
Lunch	Quick and Tasty Fajita (recipe #13) Beverage
Mid-afternoon quick energy charge	Quick Energy Charge #6 (see chapter 13)
Mid-afternoon snack	Raw vegetables, especially carrot strips
Dinner	Beef with Broccoli Stir Fry (recipe #16) Chef Salad with Raspberry Vinaigrette Dressing (recipes #34 and #38) Beverage
Evening snack/dessert	Fruit Smoothie (recipe #50)
Stretch for energy	See chapter 21 for stretches

Personal pampering	Your choice:
	   Soak in tub/whirlpool
	   Sauna/steambath
	   Manicure/pedicure
	   Facial
	   Massage
	   Get your hair done/new hairstyle

DAILY NUTRITIONAL SCORECARD
Calories: 1332

NUTRIENT	Carbohydrate	Fat	Total Protein	Animal Protein
PERCENT CALORIES	78%	10%	12%	4%
AMOUNT	273.5 G	16.5 G	44.3 G	12.3 G

Note: If you do not want to lose weight or if you are extremely active physically, you may want to increase the number of calories that you consume each day. You can do this without sacrificing your opportunity to improve your energy level if you get your additional calories from eating grains, vegetables, and fruits.

LEVEL 1: DAY 4

Before breakfast	Energy-building exercise
Breakfast	Egg White Omelette (recipe #3) Whole Wheat Toast with Jam (see Shopping List, chapter 23) Beverage
Mid-morning quick energy charge	Quick Energy Charge #7 (see chapter 15)
Mid-morning snack	Snack of your choice (see approved list)
Lunch	Hearty Vegetable Rarebit (recipe #7) Beverage
Mid-afternoon quick energy charge	Quick Energy Charge #8 (see chapter 15)
Mid-afternoon snack	Raw vegetables, especially carrot strips
Dinner	Scallops with Artichoke Sauce and Rice (recipe #25) Herbed Green Beans (recipe #30) Beverage
Evening snack/ dessert	Banana Boat (recipe #49)
Stretch for energy	See chapter 21 for stretches
Personal pampering	Your choice: Soak in tub/whirlpool Sauna/steambath Manicure/pedicure Facial Massage Get your hair done/new hairstyle

DAILY NUTRITIONAL SCORECARD
Calories: 1298

NUTRIENT	Carbohydrate	Fat	Total Protein	Animal Protein
PERCENT CALORIES	75%	7%	16%	9%
AMOUNT	250.1 G	10.4 G	53.8 G	29 G

Note: If you do not want to lose weight or if you are extremely active physically, you may want to increase the number of calories that you consume each day. You can do this without sacrificing your opportunity to improve your energy level if you get your additional calories from eating grains, vegetables, and fruits.

LEVEL 1: DAY 5

Before breakfast	Energy-building exercise
Breakfast	Oatmeal Pancakes (recipe #4, 5, or 6) Fruit Topping (recipe #43) Beverage
Mid-morning quick energy charge	Quick Energy Charge #9 (see chapter 16)
Mid-morning snack	Snack of your choice (see approved list)
Lunch	Rib-Sticking Split Pea Soup (recipe # 10) Salad Creamy Lemon Dill Dressing (recipe #39) Beverage
Mid-afternoon quick energy charge	Quick Energy Charge #10 (see chapter 17)
Mid-afternoon exercise	Energy-building exercise
Stretch for energy	See chapter 21 for stretches
Mid-afternoon snack	Raw vegetables, especially carrot strips
Dinner	Fish and Chips (recipe #24) Sweet and Sour Cabbage (recipe #31) Beverage
Evening snack/dessert	Orange-Banana Melange (recipe #46)
Stretch for energy	See chapter 21 for stretches

Personal pampering	Your choice:
	    Soak in tub/whirlpool
	    Sauna/steambath
	    Manicure/pedicure
	    Facial
	    Massage
	    Get your hair done/new hairstyle

DAILY NUTRITIONAL SCORECARD
Calories: 1268

NUTRIENT	Carbohydrate	Fat	Total Protein	Animal Protein
PERCENT CALORIES	72%	6%	22%	11%
AMOUNT	233.1 G	8.2 G	72.6 G	37.1 G

Note: If you do not want to lose weight or if you are extremely active physically, you may want to increase the number of calories that you consume each day. You can do this without sacrificing your opportunity to improve your energy level if you get your additional calories from eating grains, vegetables, and fruits.

LEVEL 1: DAY 6

Before breakfast	Energy-building exercise
Breakfast	Cold Cereal with Fruit (recipe #2) Beverage
Mid-morning quick energy charge	Quick Energy Charge #12 (see chapter 18)
Mid-morning snack	Snack of your choice (see approved list)
Lunch	Tuna Burger (recipe #9) Beverage
Mid-afternoon quick energy charge	Quick Energy Charge #16 (see chapter 22)
Mid-afternoon snack	Raw vegetables, especially carrot strips
Dinner	Zucchini Bean Casserole (recipe #19) Rice (recipe #27) Salad with Raspberry Vinaigrette Dressing (recipe #38) Beverage
Evening snack/dessert	Orange Sorbet (recipe #44)
Stretch for energy	See chapter 21 for stretches
Personal pampering	Your choice: Soak in tub/whirlpool Sauna/steambath Manicure/pedicure Facial Massage Get your hair done/new hairstyle

DAILY NUTRITIONAL SCORECARD
Calories: 1331

NUTRIENT	Carbohydrate	Fat	Total Protein	Animal Protein
PERCENT CALORIES	74%	10%	16%	8%
AMOUNT	250.3 G	14.9 G	54.9 G	25.5 G

Note: If you do not want to lose weight or if you are extremely active physically, you may want to increase the number of calories that you consume each day. You can do this without sacrificing your opportunity to improve your energy level if you get your additional calories from eating grains, vegetables, and fruits.

LEVEL 1: DAY 7

Before breakfast	Energy-building exercise
Breakfast	Hot Cereal with Raisins (recipe #1) Beverage
Mid-morning quick energy charge	Quick Energy Charge #13 (see chapter 19)
Mid-morning snack	Snack of your choice (see approved list)
Lunch	Spaghetti with Sauce and Cheese (recipe #12) Vegetable of your choice (recipe #32) Beverage
Mid-afternoon quick energy charge	Quick Energy Charge #14 (see chapter 20)
Mid-afternoon snack	Raw vegetables, especially carrot strips
Dinner	Sweet and Sour Chicken (recipe #15) Brown Rice or Noodles Beverage
Evening snack/dessert	Daniel's Jelly Roll (recipe #47)
Stretch for energy	See chapter 21 for stretches
Personal pampering	Your choice: Soak in tub/whirlpool Sauna/steambath Manicure/pedicure Facial Massage Get your hair done/new hairstyle

---

DAILY NUTRITIONAL SCORECARD
Calories: 1376

NUTRIENT	Carbohydrate	Fat	Total Protein	Animal Protein
PERCENT CALORIES	74%	8%	18%	10%
AMOUNT	253 G	12 G	60.3 G	35.8 G

Note: If you do not want to lose weight or if you are extremely active physically, you may want to increase the number of calories that you consume each day. You can do this without sacrificing your opportunity to improve your energy level if you get your additional calories from eating grains, vegetables, and fruits.

LEVEL 2: DAY 1

Before breakfast	Energy-building exercise Choose one: walking—40 minutes treadmill—30 minutes swimming—30 minutes stationary bicycle—20 minutes jogging—20 minutes
Breakfast	Hot Cereal with Raisins (recipe #1) Beverage (see recommended beverages, chapter 23)
Mid-morning quick energy charge	Quick Energy Charge #1 (see chapter 4). Quick energy charges should not be done on a full stomach; wait until your previous meal has settled.
Mid-morning snack	Snack of your choice (see recommended snacks, chapter 23)
Lunch	Spaghetti with Sauce and Cheese (recipe #12) Luncheon Salad with Pesto (recipe #33) Beverage
Mid-afternoon quick energy charge	Quick Energy Charge #2 (see chapter 6)
Mid-afternoon exercise	Energy-building exercise
Stretch for energy	See chapter 21 for stretches
Mid-afternoon snack	Raw vegetables, especially carrot strips
Personal pampering	Every day try one or more of the following suggestions for personal pampering: Soak in tub/whirlpool Sauna/steambath Manicure/pedicure Facial Massage Get your hair done/new hairstyle
Dinner	Salmon with Tomato Caper Sauce (recipe #21) Domino Potatoes (recipe #29) Herbed Green Beans (recipe #30) Beverage
Evening snack/dessert	Orange Sorbet (recipe #44)

DAILY NUTRITIONAL SCORECARD
Calories: 1282

NUTRIENT	Carbohydrate	Fat	Total Protein	Animal Protein
PERCENT CALORIES	69%	11%	17%	9%
AMOUNT	217.8 G	15 G	55.2 G	27.4 G

Note: If you do not want to lose weight or if you are extremely active physically, you may want to increase the number of calories that you consume each day. You can do this without sacrificing your opportunity to improve your energy level if you get your additional calories from eating grains, vegetables, and fruits.

LEVEL 2: DAY 2

Before breakfast	Energy-building exercise
Breakfast	Cold Cereal with Fruit (recipe #2) Beverage
Mid-morning quick energy charge	Quick Energy Charge #3 (see chapter 7)
Mid-morning snack	Snack of your choice (See approved list in chapter 23)
Lunch	Double Decker Sandwich (recipe #8) Beverage
Mid-afternoon quick energy charge	Quick Energy Charge #4 (see chapter 9)
Mid-afternoon exercise	Energy-building exercise
Stretch for energy	See chapter 21 for stretches
Mid-afternoon snack	Raw vegetables, especially carrot strips
Personal pampering	Your choice: Soak in tub/whirlpool Sauna/steambath Manicure/pedicure Facial Massage Get your hair done/new hairstyle
Dinner	Fish and Chips (recipe #24) Sweet and Tangy Carrots (recipe #28) Beverage
Evening snack/dessert	Baked Apple with Raisins (recipe #48)

DAILY NUTRITIONAL SCORECARD
Calories: 1203

NUTRIENT	Carbohydrate	Fat	Total Protein	Animal Protein
PERCENT CALORIES	74%	7%	19%	11%
AMOUNT	227 G	9.3 G	59.9 G	32.3 G

Note: If you do not want to lose weight or if you are extremely active physically, you may want to increase the number of calories that you consume each day. You can do this without sacrificing your opportunity to improve your energy level if you get your additional calories from eating grains, vegetables, and fruits.

LEVEL 2: DAY 3

Before breakfast	Energy-building exercise
Breakfast	Cold Cereal with Fruit (recipe #2) Beverage
Mid-morning quick energy charge	Quick Energy Charge #5 (see chapter 12)
Mid-morning snack	Snack of your choice (see approved list)
Lunch	Tuna Burger (recipe #9) Beverage
Mid-afternoon quick energy charge	Quick Energy Charge #6 (see chapter 13)
Mid-afternoon exercise	Energy-building exercise
Stretch for energy	See chapter 21 for stretches
Mid-afternoon snack	Raw vegetables, especially carrot strips
Personal pampering	Your choice: Soak in tub/whirlpool Sauna/steambath Manicure/pedicure Facial Massage Get your hair done/new hairstyle
Dinner	Vegetable Lasagna (recipe #17) Salad Creamy Lemon Dill Dressing (recipe #39) Beverage
Evening snack/dessert	Fruit Smoothie (recipe #50)

DAILY NUTRITIONAL SCORECARD
Calories: 1210

NUTRIENT	Carbohydrate	Fat	Total Protein	Animal Protein
PERCENT CALORIES	73%	9%	17%	6%
AMOUNT	224.8 G	11.8 G	51.3 G	18.3 G

Note: If you do not want to lose weight or if you are extremely active physically, you may want to increase the number of calories that you consume each day. You can do this without sacrificing your opportunity to improve your energy level if you get your additional calories from eating grains, vegetables, and fruits.

LEVEL 2: DAY 4

Before breakfast	Energy-building exercise
Breakfast	Egg White Omelette (recipe #3) Whole-Wheat Toast with Jam (see approved list) Beverage
Mid-morning quick energy charge	Quick Energy Charge #7 (see chapter 15)
Mid-morning snack	Snack of your choice (see approved list)
Lunch	Rib-Sticking Split Pea Soup (recipe #10) Luncheon Salad with Pesto (recipe #33) Beverage
Mid-afternoon quick energy charge	Quick Energy Charge #8 (see chapter 15)
Mid-afternoon exercise	Energy-building exercise
Stretch for energy	See chapter 21 for stretches
Mid-afternoon snack	Raw vegetables, especially carrot strips
Personal pampering	Your choice: Soak in tub/whirlpool Sauna/steambath Manicure/pedicure Facial Massage Get your hair done/new hairstyle
Dinner	Zucchini Bean Casserole (recipe #19) Salad Raspberry Vinaigrette Dressing (recipe #38) Beverage
Evening snack/dessert	Orange Banana Melange (recipe #46)

DAILY NUTRITIONAL SCORECARD
Calories: 1255

NUTRIENT	Carbohydrate	Fat	Total Protein	Animal Protein
PERCENT CALORIES	72%	9%	19%	9%
AMOUNT	229.6 G	12.2 G	61.4 G	27.2 G

Note: If you do not want to lose weight or if you are extremely active physically, you may want to increase the number of calories that you consume each day. You can do this without sacrificing your opportunity to improve your energy level if you get your additional calories from eating grains, vegetables, and fruits.

LEVEL 2: DAY 5

Before breakfast	Energy-building exercise
Breakfast	Hot Cereal with Raisins (recipe #1) Beverage
Mid-morning quick energy charge	Quick Energy Charge #9 (see chapter 16)
Mid-morning snack	Snack of your choice (see approved list in chapter 23)
Lunch	Quinoa-Tomato Soup (recipe #11) Luncheon Salad with Pesto (recipe #33) Beverage
Mid-afternoon quick energy charge	Quick Energy Charge #10 (see chapter 17)
Mid-afternoon exercise	Energy-building exercise
Stretch for energy	See chapter 21 for stretches
Mid-afternoon snack	Raw vegetables, especially carrot strips
Personal pampering	Your choice: Soak in tub/whirlpool Sauna/steambath Manicure/pedicure Facial Massage Get your hair done/new hairstyle
Dinner	Chicken with Fettucine (recipe #14) Spinach with Feta Cheese (recipe #26) Beverage
Evening snack/dessert	Banana Boat (recipe #49)

DAILY NUTRITIONAL SCORECARD
Calories: 1231

NUTRIENT	Carbohydrate	Fat	Total Protein	Animal Protein
PERCENT CALORIES	67%	11%	21%	10%
AMOUNT	204.7 G	14.3 G	65.2 G	30.7 G

Note: If you do not want to lose weight or if you are extremely active physically, you may want to increase the number of calories that you consume each day. You can do this without sacrificing your opportunity to improve your energy level if you get your additional calories from eating grains, vegetables, and fruits.

LEVEL 2: DAY 6

Before breakfast	Energy-building exercise
Breakfast	Oatmeal Pancakes (recipe #4, 5, or 6) Fruit Topping (recipe #43) Beverage
Mid-morning quick energy charge	Quick Energy Charge #12 (see chapter 18)
Mid-morning snack	Snack of your choice (see approved list in chapter 23)
Lunch	Hearty Vegetable Rarebit (recipe #7) Beverage
Mid-afternoon quick energy charge	Quick Energy Charge #14 (see chapter 20)
Mid-afternoon exercise	Energy-building exercise
Stretch for energy	See chapter 21 for stretches
Mid-afternoon snack	Raw vegetables, especially carrot strips

Personal pampering	Your choice:
	    Soak in tub/whirlpool
	    Sauna/steambath
	    Manicure/pedicure
	    Facial
	    Massage
	    Get your hair done/new hairstyle

Dinner	Scallops with Artichoke Sauce and Rice (recipe #25) Vegetable of your choice (recipe #32) Beverage
Evening snack/dessert	Two California Orbap Cookies (recipe #45)

DAILY NUTRITIONAL SCORECARD
Calories: 1233*

NUTRIENT	Carbohydrate	Fat	Total Protein	Animal Protein
PERCENT CALORIES	72%	8%	18%	8%
AMOUNT	227.5 G	11.2 G	55 G	25.1 G

Note: If you do not want to lose weight or if you are extremely active physically, you may want to increase the number of calories that you consume each day. You can do this without sacrificing your opportunity to improve your energy level if you get your additional calories from eating grains, vegetables, and fruits.

LEVEL 2: DAY 7

Before breakfast	Energy-building exercise
Breakfast	Cold Cereal with Fruit (recipe #2) Beverage
Mid-morning quick energy charge	Quick Energy Charge #16 (see chapter 22)
Mid-morning snack	Snack of your choice (see approved list)
Lunch	Two Quick and Tasty Fajitas (recipe #13) Beverage
Mid-afternoon quick energy charge	Quick Energy Charge #14 (see chapter 20)
Mid-afternoon exercise	Energy-building exercise
Stretch for energy	See chapter 21 for stretches
Mid-afternoon snack	Raw vegetables, especially carrot strips
Personal pampering	Your choice: Soak in tub/whirlpool Sauna/steambath Manicure/pedicure Facial Massage Get your hair done/new hairstyle
Dinner	Potato Pancakes with Applesauce (recipe #18) Sweet and Sour Cabbage (recipe #31) Beverage
Evening snack/dessert	Daniel's Jelly Roll (recipe #47)

DAILY NUTRITIONAL SCORECARD
Calories: 1241

NUTRIENT	Carbohydrate	Fat	Total Protein	Animal Protein
PERCENT CALORIES	81%	7%	12%	2%
AMOUNT	257.9 G	10.3 G	38.1 G	7.3 G

Note: If you do not want to lose weight or if you are extremely active physically, you may want to increase the number of calories that you consume each day. You can do this without sacrificing your opportunity to improve your energy level if you get your additional calories from eating grains, vegetables, and fruits.

LEVEL 3: DAY 1

Before breakfast	Energy-building exercise Choose one: walking—40 minutes treadmill—30 minutes swimming—30 minutes stationary bicycle—20 minutes jogging—20 minutes
Breakfast	Hot Cereal with Raisins (recipe #1) Beverage (see recommended beverages, chapter 23)
Mid-morning quick energy charge	Quick Energy Charge #1 (see chapter 4) Wait until your previous meal has settled.
Mid-morning exercise	Energy-building exercise
Mid-morning snack	Apple or pear
Lunch	Spaghetti with Sauce and Cheese (recipe #12) Salad Raspberry Vinaigrette Dressing (recipe #38) Beverage
Mid-afternoon quick energy charge	Quick Energy Charge #2 (see chapter 6)
Mid-afternoon exercise	Energy-building exercise
Stretch for energy	See chapter 21 for stretches
Mid-afternoon snack	Raw vegetables, especially carrot strips
Personal pampering	Every day try one or more of the following suggestions for personal pampering: Soak in tub/whirlpool Sauna/steambath Manicure/pedicure Facial Massage Get your hair done/new hairstyle
Dinner	Poached Fish with Sauce (recipe #23) Herbed Green Beans (recipe #30) Vegetable of your choice (recipe #32) Beverage
Evening snack/dessert	Banana Boat (recipe #49)

DAILY NUTRITIONAL SCORECARD
Calories: 1227

NUTRIENT	Carbohydrate	Fat	Total Protein	Animal Protein
PERCENT CALORIES	69%	10%	21%	11%
AMOUNT	212 G	13 G	63.4 G	33.2 G

Note: If you do not want to lose weight or if you are extremely active physically, you may want to increase the number of calories that you consume each day. You can do this without sacrificing your opportunity to improve your energy level if you get your additional calories from eating grains, vegetables, and fruits.

LEVEL 3: DAY 2

Before breakfast	Energy-building exercise
Breakfast	Hot Cereal with Raisins (recipe #1) Beverage
Mid-morning quick energy charge	Quick Energy Charge #3 (see chapter 7)
Mid-morning exercise	Energy-building exercise
Mid-morning snack	Snack of your choice (see approved list)
Lunch	Double Decker Sandwich (recipe #8) Beverage
Mid-afternoon quick energy charge	Quick Energy Charge #4 (see chapter 9)
Mid-afternoon exercise	Energy-building exercise
Stretch for energy	See chapter 21 for stretches
Mid-afternoon snack	Raw vegetables, especially carrot strips

Personal pampering	Your choice:
	    Soak in tub/whirlpool
	    Sauna/steambath
	    Manicure/pedicure
	    Facial
	    Massage
	    Get your hair done/new hairstyle

Dinner	Salmon with Tomato Caper Sauce (recipe #21) Domino Potatoes (recipe #29) Beverage
Evening snack/dessert	Orange Sorbet (recipe #44)

DAILY NUTRITIONAL SCORECARD
Calories: 1193

NUTRIENT	Carbohydrate	Fat	Total Protein	Animal Protein
PERCENT CALORIES	69%	9%	18%	8%
AMOUNT	207.7 G	12.5 G	52.5 G	22.7 G

Note: If you do not want to lose weight or if you are extremely active physically, you may want to increase the number of calories that you consume each day. You can do this without sacrificing your opportunity to improve your energy level if you get your additional calories from eating grains, vegetables, and fruits.

LEVEL 3: DAY 3

Before breakfast	Energy-building exercise
Breakfast	Egg-white omelette (recipe #3) English muffin with jam (see approved list) Beverage
Mid-morning quick energy charge	Quick Energy Charge #5 (see chapter 12)
Mid-morning exercise	Energy-building exercise
Mid-morning snack	Snack of your choice (see approved list)
Lunch	Rib-Sticking Split Pea Soup (recipe #10) Luncheon Salad with Pesto (recipe #35) Beverage
Mid-afternoon quick energy charge	Quick Energy Charge #6 (see chapter 13)
Mid-afternoon exercise	Energy-building exercise
Stretch for energy	See chapter 21 for stretches
Mid-afternoon snack	Raw vegetables, especially carrot strips

Personal pampering	Your choice:
	    Soak in tub/whirlpool
	    Sauna/steambath
	    Manicure/pedicure
	    Facial
	    Massage
	    Get your hair done/new hairstyle

Dinner	Baked Potato San Diego Chili (recipe #20) Salad Creamy Lemon Dill Dressing (recipe #39) Beverage
Evening snack/dessert	Baked Apple with Raisins (recipe #48)

DAILY NUTRITIONAL SCORECARD
Calories: 1193

NUTRIENT	Carbohydrate	Fat	Total Protein	Animal Protein
PERCENT CALORIES	80%	4%	16%	3%
AMOUNT	241.6 G	5.8 G	49 G	10.2 G

Note: If you do not want to lose weight or if you are extremely active physically, you may want to increase the number of calories that you consume each day. You can do this without sacrificing your opportunity to improve your energy level if you get your additional calories from eating grains, vegetables, and fruits.

LEVEL 3: DAY 4

Before breakfast	Energy-building exercise
Breakfast	Hot Cereal with Raisins (recipe #1) Beverage
Mid-morning quick energy charge	Quick Energy Charge #7 (see chapter 15)
Mid-morning exercise	Energy-building exercise
Mid-morning snack	Snack of your choice (see approved list)
Lunch	Tuna Burger (recipe #9) Beverage
Mid-afternoon quick energy charge	Quick Energy Charge #8 (see chapter 15)
Mid-afternoon exercise	Energy-building exercise
Stretch for energy	See chapter 21 for stretches
Mid-afternoon snack	Raw vegetables, especially carrot strips
Personal pampering	Your choice: Soak in tub/whirlpool Sauna/steambath Manicure/pedicure Facial Massage Get your hair done/new hairstyle
Dinner	Potato Pancakes with Applesauce (recipe #18) Sweet and Tangy Carrots (recipe #28) Beverage
Evening snack/dessert	Fruit Smoothie (recipe #50)

DAILY NUTRITIONAL SCORECARD
Calories: 1238

NUTRIENT	Carbohydrate	Fat	Total Protein	Animal Protein
PERCENT CALORIES	78%	8%	14%	3%
AMOUNT	241.8 G	10.9 G	43.3 G	9 G

Note: If you do not want to lose weight or if you are extremely active physically, you may want to increase the number of calories that you consume each day. You can do this without sacrificing your opportunity to improve your energy level if you get your additional calories from eating grains, vegetables, and fruits.

LEVEL 3: DAY 5

Before breakfast	Energy-building exercise
Breakfast	Oatmeal Pancakes (recipe #4, 5, or 6) Fruit Topping (recipe #43) Beverage
Mid-morning quick energy charge	Quick Energy Charge #9 (see chapter 16)
Mid-morning exercise	Energy-building exercise
Mid-morning snack	Snack of your choice (see approved list)
Lunch	Quinoa-Tomato Soup (recipe #11) Raw vegetables (e.g., carrots, celery, cucumber spears) Spicy Vegetable Dip (recipe #36) Beverage
Mid-afternoon quick energy charge	Quick Energy Charge #10 (see chapter 17)
Mid-afternoon exercise	Energy-building exercise
Stretch for energy	See chapter 21 for stretches
Mid-afternoon snack	Raw vegetables, especially carrot strips
Personal pampering	Your choice: Soak in tub/whirlpool Sauna/steambath Manicure/pedicure Facial Massage Get your hair done/new hairstyle
Dinner	Delicious Fish Stew (recipe #22) Salad Raspberry Vinaigrette Dressing (recipe #38) Beverage
Evening snack/dessert	Banana Boat (recipe #49)

DAILY NUTRITIONAL SCORECARD
Calories: 1044

NUTRIENT	Carbohydrate	Fat	Total Protein	Animal Protein
PERCENT CALORIES	74%	9%	17%	8%
AMOUNT	194.7 G	10 G	45.6 G	21.2 G

Note: If you do not want to lose weight or if you are extremely active physically, you may want to increase the number of calories that you consume each day. You can do this without sacrificing your opportunity to improve your energy level if you get your additional calories from eating grains, vegetables, and fruits.

LEVEL 3: DAY 6

Before breakfast	Energy-building exercise
Breakfast	Hot Cereal with Raisins (recipe #1) Beverage
Mid-morning quick energy charge	Quick Energy Charge #11 (see chapter 17)
Mid-morning exercise	Energy-building exercise
Mid-morning snack	Snack of your choice (see approved list)
Lunch	Hearty Vegetable Rarebit (recipe #7) Beverage
Mid-afternoon quick energy charge	Quick Energy Charge #12 (see chapter 18)
Mid-afternoon exercise	Energy-building exercise
Stretch for energy	See chapter 21 for stretches
Mid-afternoon snack	Raw vegetables, especially carrot strips
Personal pampering	Your choice: Soak in tub/whirlpool Sauna/steambath Manicure/pedicure Facial Massage Get your hair done/new hairstyle
Dinner	Vegetable Lasagna (recipe #17) Spinach with Feta Cheese (recipe #26) Beverage
Evening snack/dessert	Baked Apple with Raisins (recipe #48)

DAILY NUTRITIONAL SCORECARD
Calories: 1144

NUTRIENT	Carbohydrate	Fat	Total Protein	Animal Protein
PERCENT CALORIES	76%	9%	14%	3%
AMOUNT	220.7 G	12 G	41.5 G	9 G

Note: If you do not want to lose weight or if you are extremely active physically, you may want to increase the number of calories that you consume each day. You can do this without sacrificing your opportunity to improve your energy level if you get your additional calories from eating grains, vegetables, and fruits.

LEVEL 3: DAY 7

Before breakfast	Energy-building exercise
Breakfast	Cold Cereal with Fruit (recipe #2) Beverage
Mid-morning quick energy charge	Quick Energy Charge #13 (see chapter 19)
Mid-morning exercise	Energy-building exercise
Mid-morning snack	Snack of your choice (see approved list)
Lunch	Quick and Tasty Fajita (recipe #13) Beverage
Mid-afternoon quick energy charge	Quick Energy Charge #14 (see chapter 20)
Mid-afternoon exercise	Energy-building exercise
Stretch for energy	See chapter 21 for stretches
Mid-afternoon snack	Raw vegetables, especially carrot strips

Personal pampering	Your choice:
	    Soak in tub/whirlpool
	    Sauna/steambath
	    Manicure/pedicure
	    Facial
	    Massage
	    Get your hair done/new hairstyle

Dinner	Zucchini Bean Casserole (recipe #19) Sweet and Sour Cabbage (recipe #31) Beverage
Evening snack/dessert	Baked Raspberry Pear (recipe #51)

DAILY NUTRITIONAL SCORECARD
Calories: 1114

NUTRIENT	Carbohydrate	Fat	Total Protein	Animal Protein
PERCENT CALORIES	75%	11%	14%	6%
AMOUNT	224.6 G	14 G	41 G	18 G

Note: If you do not want to lose weight or if you are extremely active physically, you may want to increase the number of calories that you consume each day. You can do this without sacrificing your opportunity to improve your energy level if you get your additional calories from eating grains, vegetables, and fruits.

Chapter 11

High-Energy Food Supplements

This chapter offers information about supplements used to protect you from psychological and physical stress and suggests ways you can augment your body's ability to function more efficiently. You will learn:

- What antistress vitamins and minerals can do for you. You will also learn their recommended daily allowances, possible side effects of overdoses, and symptoms of deficiency.
- Natural sources of high-energy, antistress vitamins and minerals.

WARNING: *Do not take food supplements without the approval of your physician or a qualified nutritionist.*

NUTRITIONAL SUPPLEMENTS AND ENERGY

Think of vitamins and minerals as the catalysts that make your system work better. Just as a car's engine will run rough on gasoline that lacks the right combination of catalysts, your body will not burn its fuel efficiently without these essential ingredients. The result is that you will not have as much energy. You will run sluggishly.

The issue then is not whether or not you should have vitamins and minerals in your diet. The issue is from where you should get them. Even after many years of investigation we still have a long way to go before we can resolve this issue with any certainty. Theoretically, no one who eats a balanced diet should require vitamin or mineral supplements. Yet millions of vitamins and minerals are sold every day to people who seek to replace vanishing natural sources of energy. The following chart outlines some of the various ways we are losing those natural sources:

HOW OUR ENVIRONMENT DEPRIVES YOU OF
NATURAL SOURCES OF ENERGY

Problem	Cause	Resulting Energy Loss
Depleted soil	Poor agricultural methods Poor land management	Food deficient in important nutrients
Refined foods	Processing to make food last longer	Food depleted of optimal nutrients
Food not fresh	Food shipped coast to coast and/or sold long after the optimal freshness date	Nutritional content depleted
Pollution	Result of industrialization: polluted water, soil, air	Toxins in the environment as well as in the food
Food additives/ chemicals in food	Preservatives, waxes, fertilizers, fungicides, pesticides, coloring agents, artificial flavorings	Body can't process food properly
Stress	Diverse sources, ranging from fast pace of modern world to work problems to environmental noise	Body robbed of essential nutrients

Fortunately, evidence has been mounting to show that vitamin and mineral supplements *can* protect you from the effects of an increasingly hostile environment. We like to think of a supplementation program as an insurance policy. Healthy people probably can take a high-quality multivitamin without supervision. Anything beyond that requires medical/nutritional supervision by a professional. We urge you to consult a qualified nutritionist to help you pinpoint your individual supplementation needs.

ANTISTRESS VITAMINS

Vitamins soluble in water are used up rapidly by the body when it is under stress. Ironically, these same vitamins are the ones you need most when the going gets tough! B vitamins are often included in anti-stress formulas.

Warning: Any B vitamin taken out of proportion to all other B vitamins, or taken alone, can cause depletion and symptoms of deficiency in all the other B vitamins, since they are excreted along with the excess of the one you are supplementing. In other words, if you took only B_1 without the other B vitamins, you would get the deficiency symptoms of all of the B vitamins you are not taking. *Always take all the B vitamins together in a balanced formula.*

Don't fool around with your own combination of B vitamins. Eat a variety of natural foods that are rich in these vitamins.

VITAMIN B_1: THIAMINE

Thiamine is known as the anti-aging vitamin. It is essential for metabolizing protein and converting glucose into energy. Appropriate amounts of B_1 increase your stamina and prevent fatigue. Thiamine

- Protects the heart muscle
- Promotes growth
- Helps develop muscle tone in the stomach and intestines
- Helps relieve constipation and aids digestion and peristalsis
- Helps prevent fluid retention
- Protects against the effects of lead poisoning

Vitamin B_1 helps rid your body of acids formed when glucose is converted into energy. Otherwise the acid by-products of sugar breakdown can result in an accumulation of toxic acids in the brain, acid irritation of the heart muscle, and nerve cell damage. Severe B_1 deficiency can cause beriberi, neuritis, and edema.

FACTS ABOUT VITAMIN B_1 (THIAMINE)

Solubility: Water
Minimum Daily Requirement: 1–1.5 mg.

Symptoms of Deficiency	Symptoms of Overdose	Things That Use Up the Vitamin Too Fast
Loss of appetite	Same as the symptoms of B-complex deficiency. (See warning note at beginning of chapter.)	Alcohol
Slow heartbeat		Tobacco
Chronic constipation		Coffee
Irritability		Sugar
Diabetes		Processed food
Depression		Raw clams
Nervous exhaustion		Refined foods
Poor lactation		
Intestinal disorders		
Gastric disorders		
Forgetfulness		
Fatigue		
Shortness of breath		
Pain sensitivity		

Thiamine exists in a wide variety of plant and animal food sources, but as part of your effort to eliminate fat and reduce cholesterol, you should rely mainly on vegetarian sources.

NATURAL FOOD SOURCES OF VITAMIN B₁ (THIAMINE)

Vegetarian	Animal*
Asparagus	**Lacto**
Brewer's yeast	
Cabbage	Cheese
Carrots	Yogurt
Celery	Milk
Coconuts	
Grapefruit	**Meat**
Lemons	Organ meats
Nuts	Pork
Parsley	
Pineapple	
Radishes	
Rice polishings	
Seeds	
Wheat germ	
Wheat bran	
Whole-grain cereals	
Watercress	

*Not recommended

VITAMIN B₂: RIBOFLAVIN

Riboflavin might be called the anti-cataract vitamin. It is essential for growth, healthy eyes, and general well-being. Riboflavin also

- Promotes healthy skin, nails, and hair
- Improves thyroid function
- Is essential for oxidation and energy release
- Helps metabolize protein and assimilate iron

Early signs of deficiency are sores around the mouth, sensitivity to light, and lack of stamina.

FACTS ABOUT VITAMIN B$_2$ (RIBOFLAVIN)

Solubility: Water
Minimum Daily Requirement: 1.3–1.7 mg.

Symptoms of Deficiency	Symptoms of Overdose	Things That Use Up the Vitamin Too Fast
Light sensitivity	Same as the symptoms of B-complex defi-	Alcohol
Lack of stamina	ciency. (See warning note at beginning of	Tobacco
Digestive disturbances	chapter.)	Coffee
Cataracts		Sugar
Hair loss		Refined foods
Depression		
Sore and red tongue		
Bloodshot eyes		

Like vitamin B$_1$, B$_2$ is water-soluble. The excess beyond what your body needs is excreted in urine and does not normally build up. A toxic dose for vitamin B$_2$ has not yet been identified. Remember, always take B vitamins together in a balanced formula. B$_2$ is present in many plant and animal sources. As part of your effort to eliminate fat and reduce cholesterol, you should rely mainly on vegetarian sources of vitamin B$_2$.

NATURAL FOOD SOURCES OF VITAMIN B$_2$
(RIBOFLAVIN)

Vegetarian	Animal*
Apples	**Lacto**
Apricots	
Blackstrap molasses	Cheese
Brewer's yeast	Yogurt
Cabbage	Milk
Carrots	
Coconuts	**Meat**
Collards	
Dandelion greens	Organ meats
Grapefruit	Pork
Prunes	
Spinach	
Turnip greens	
Whole-grain cereals	
Watercress	

*Not recommended

VITAMIN B₃: NIACIN

Niacin, often called the anti-pellagra vitamin, is essential for healthy functioning of the nervous system and for proper circulation. It is believed to help prevent migraine headaches and maintain healthy skin. Niacin is a key factor in

- Metabolizing protein, fat, and carbohydrate
- Helping to reduce cholesterol levels
- Helping to prevent fatigue

Niacin also goes by other names: niacinamide, nicotinic acid, and nicotinic acidomide. The amount required varies from one person to another.

FACTS ABOUT VITAMIN B₃ (NIACIN)

Solubility: Water
Minimum Daily Requirement: 10–13 mg.

Symptoms of Deficiency	Symptoms of Overdose	Things That Use Up the Vitamin Too Fast
Unpleasant mouth odor	Red, prickly skin, liver damage, stomach ulcers, jaundice. (See previous warning note.)	Alcohol
Psychological imbalance		Corn
Canker sores		Coffee
Appetite loss		Sugar
Depression, fatigue		Processed foods
Headaches		Refined foods
Indigestion		Antibiotics
Insomnia		
Nausea		
Skin eruptions		
Muscular weakness		

Just like B₁, B₃ is water-soluble. But scientists have found that massive doses of B₃ can cause severe liver damage, peptic ulcers, and diabetes. The individual daily requirement for niacin is considerably higher than that of the other B vitamins. Remember to take B vitamins together in a balanced formula.

Vitamin B₃ can be found in many plant and animal sources. As part of your effort to eliminate fat and reduce cholesterol, you should rely mainly on vegetarian sources.

NATURAL FOOD SOURCES OF VITAMIN B₃
(NIACIN)

Vegetarian	Animal*
Brewer's yeast	**Lacto/Ovo**
Brown rice	
Green vegetables	Milk products
Nuts	Eggs
Peanuts	
Rice bran	**Meat**
Rhubarb	Fish
Soybeans	Liver
Sunflower seeds	Poultry
Torula yeast	
Wheat germ	
Whole-wheat products	

*Not recommended

VITAMIN B₅: PANTOTHENIC ACID

Pantothenic acid could be called the energy or antistress B vitamin. It is essential for the body's proper use of sugar and fat for energy. As mental or physical stress increases, the body demands increasing amounts of stress-protective pantothenic acid. B₅ also

- Prevents wrinkles and premature aging
- Stimulates the adrenal glands
- Maintains an appropriate level of blood sugar
- Increases energy and vitality
- Helps ward off infections
- Plays a key part in ensuring a speedy recovery from illness

Pantothenic acid also has been used to treat allergies, arthritis, low blood sugar, baldness, and tooth decay.

FACTS ABOUT VITAMIN B₅ (PANTOTHENIC ACID)

Solubility: Water
Minimum Daily Requirement: Not established
(estimates: 4–50 mg.)

Symptoms of Deficiency	Symptoms of Overdose	Things That Use Up the Vitamin Too Fast
Low stress resistance	Same symptoms as B-complex deficiency.	Alcohol
Gray hair	(See remarks below and previous warning.)	Tobacco
Stomach distress		Coffee
Allergies, asthma		Sugar
Hair loss		Stress
Depression		
Sore and burning feet		
Low blood sugar		
Muscle cramps		
Low blood pressure		
Irritability		
Duodenal ulcer		
Diarrhea		

Scientists have found no normally occurring cases of pantothenic acid deficiency. Like vitamin B₁, pantothenic acid is water-soluble and is excreted in urine. Scientists have not yet identified the toxic dose for vitamin B₅. Remember, always take B vitamins together in a balanced formula.

Vitamin B₅ comes from many plant and animal sources. As part of the effort to eliminate fat and reduce cholesterol, you should rely mainly on vegetarian sources of B₅.

NATURAL FOOD SOURCES OF VITAMIN B₅
(PANTOTHENIC ACID)

Vegetarian	Animal*
Beans	**Ovo**
Blackstrap molasses	
Brewer's yeast	Egg Yolk
Cauliflower	
Green vegetables	**Meat**
Mushrooms	
Peas	Liver
Peanuts	Kidneys
Wheat bran	Salmon
Wheat germ	
Whole grains	
*Not recommended	

VITAMIN B$_6$: PYRIDOXINE

Pyridoxine, the "tranquilizer" vitamin, is essential in activating many of the body's enzymes and enzyme systems and in the production of antibodies to protect you from bacterial diseases. It is also essential to DNA and RNA synthesis. There is some evidence B$_6$ may help prevent bladder cancer. It also

- Helps promote digestion and prevent skin disorders
- Protects against tooth decay
- Helps your body maintain a good sodium-potassium balance
- Is effective against insomnia

Vitamin B$_6$ has been used in the treatment of Parkinson's disease, arthritic and rheumatic conditions, mental retardation, sexual disorders, pancreatitis, and hypoglycemia.

FACTS ABOUT VITAMIN B$_6$ (PYRIDOXINE)

Solubility: Water
Minimum Daily Requirement: 2.0–2.5 mg.

Symptoms of Deficiency	Symptoms of Overdose	Things That Use Up the Vitamin Too Fast
Acne, skin disorders	Doses of 150 mg. can cause sleepiness. Daily doses over 200 mg. have caused a dependency state after withdrawal. (See remarks below and previous warning note.)	Alcohol
Anemia		Tobacco
Arthritis		Coffee
Irritability		Birth-control pills
Hair loss		Radiation exposure
Depression		
Learning disabilities		
Weakness		
Sore mouth and lips		
Bad breath		
Tooth decay		
Migraine headaches		
Premature senility		

B$_6$ is another of the water-soluble vitamins, so excess B$_6$ is excreted in urine. Scientists have not yet identified the toxic dose for vitamin B$_6$. Remember, always take B vitamins together in a balanced formula.

B$_6$ can be found in many plant and animal sources. As part of your effort to eliminate fat and reduce cholesterol, you should rely mainly on vegetarian sources of B$_6$.

NATURAL FOOD SOURCES OF VITAMIN B$_6$
(PYRIDOXINE)

Vegetarian	Animal*
Avocados	**Lacto/Ovo**
Bananas	
Blackstrap molasses	Milk
Brewer's yeast	Egg yolks
Cabbage	
Cantaloupe	**Meat**
Carrots	Desiccated liver
Green leafy vegetables	Fish
Green peppers	Organ meats
Peanuts	
Pecans	
Prunes	
Raisins	
Soybeans	
Walnuts	
Wheat bran	
Wheat germ	
Whole grains	

*Not recommended

BIOTIN

Biotin helps to metabolize fats and protein and is necessary for the utilization of pantothenic acid. It helps your body
- Use B-complex vitamins
- Is essential for cell growth
- Promotes hair growth and helps prevent baldness

Your body can produce biotin in your intestines if enough friendly bacteria are present there. Biotin deficiencies occur if one eats raw egg whites in large amounts (about twenty per day).

FACTS ABOUT BIOTIN

Solubility: Water
Minimum Daily Requirement: 150–300 mcg.

Symptoms of Deficiency	Symptoms of Overdose	Things That Use Up the Vitamin Too Fast
Dry skin	Actual toxic dose unknown. Biotin overdose would have the same symptoms as vitamin B-complex deficiency. (See remarks below and previous warning note.)	Alcohol
Depression		Coffee
Fatigue		Raw egg whites
Poor appetite		Sugar
Lack of stamina		Antibiotics
Eczema		Refined food
Hair loss		Processed food
Dandruff		
Seborrhea		
Lung infections		
Heart abnormalities		
Drowsiness		
Hallucinations		
Anemia		

Like B_1, Biotin is water-soluble and any excess is excreted in urine. No toxic dose for biotin has yet been identified. Always take B vitamins together in a balanced formula.

Biotin can be obtained from both plant and animal sources. As part of your effort to eliminate fat and reduce cholesterol, you should rely mainly on vegetarian sources.

NATURAL FOOD SOURCES OF BIOTIN

Vegetarian	Animal*
Beans	**Lacto/Ovo**
Brewer's yeast	
Mushrooms	Milk
Peanuts	Egg yolks
Soybeans	Yogurt
Unpolished rice	
Whole grains	**Meat**
	Liver
	Kidneys

*Not recommended

VITAMIN B_9: FOLIC ACID

Folic acid could be called the healing vitamin, as it helps build antibodies that prevent and heal infections. Folic acid works with B_{12} to help form red blood cells. It also works with B_{12} and vitamin C to help your body break down and use proteins. It has been found to help prevent premature gray hair. It is essential to cell reproduction.

Folic acid enables the body to utilize amino acids and sugar. A deficiency of B_9 leads to serious skin disorders, impaired circulation, and loss of hair.

FACTS ABOUT VITAMIN B_9 (FOLIC ACID)

Solubility: Water
Minimum Daily Requirement: 400 mcg.

Symptoms of Deficiency	Symptoms of Overdose	Things That Use Up the Vitamin Too Fast
Hair loss	Actual toxic dose unknown. A B_9 overdose would have the same symptoms as a vitamin B-complex deficiency. (See remarks below and the previous warning.)	Alcohol
Serious skin disorders		Coffee
Impaired circulation		Tobacco
Mental depression		Sugar
Anemia		Stress
Fatigue		Refined food
Graying hair		Processed food
Digestion problems		Heat (cooking)
Insomnia		Sulfa drugs
Tongue inflammation		Fever
Memory problems		Birth-control pills
Reproduction problems		
Walking problems		
Speaking problems		

Like B_1, folic acid is water-soluble and any excess is excreted in urine. Scientists have not yet identified the toxic dose for folic acid. Always take B vitamins together in a balanced formula.

Folic acid can be found in many foods. As part of your effort to eliminate and reduce cholesterol, you should rely mainly on vegetarian sources of B_9.

NATURAL FOOD SOURCES OF VITAMIN B$_9$
(FOLIC ACID)

Vegetarian	Animal*
Asparagus	**Lacto/Ovo**
Broccoli	
Dates	Milk
Grapefruit	Egg
Green leafy vegetables	Yogurt
Lettuce	
Lima beans	**Meat**
Mushrooms	
Nuts	Liver
Oranges	Oysters
Peanuts	Salmon
White potatoes	Tuna
Spinach	
Whole grains	

*Not recommended

VITAMIN B$_{12}$: COBALAMIN

Cobalamin is known as the red vitamin. It is essential to the regeneration and production of the red blood cells. Cobalamin or cyanocobalamin is also important for proper nerve functioning, helping to maintain the nerve sheath so that it can transmit messages. Vitamin B$_{12}$

- Promotes a healthy appetite
- Prevents anemia
- Promotes growth in children
- Is essential for blood-cell growth and longevity

FACTS ABOUT VITAMIN B$_{12}$ (COBALAMIN)

Solubility: Water
Minimum Daily Requirement: 1–5 mcg.

Symptoms of Deficiency	Symptoms of Overdose	Things That Use Up the Vitamin Too Fast
Impaired reflexes	Actual toxic dose unknown. B$_{12}$ overdose	Alcohol
Depression	would have the same symptoms as the	Coffee
Fatigue	vitamin B-complex deficiency. (See	Calcium deficiency
Pernicious anemia	remarks below and the previous warning.)	B$_6$ deficiency

Symptoms of Deficiency	Symptoms of Overdose	Things That Use Up the Vitamin Too Fast
Weakness in legs/arms		Tobacco
Walking difficulties		Liver disease
Speaking difficulties		Processed food
Memory loss		Laxatives
Nervousness		
Poor concentration		
Sore mouth		
Poor appetite in children		

Like vitamin B_1, B_{12} is water-soluble and the excess beyond what your body needs is excreted in urine. Science has not yet identified the toxic dose for cobalamin. Always take B vitamins together in a balanced formula.

Your body can produce vitamin B_{12} in the intestines if there is a sufficient amount of microflora available. Some nutritionists question whether enough B_{12} can be provided this way and claim that strict vegetarians who use no animal products will begin to show deficiency symptoms within five or six years, when the B_{12} stored in the liver is used up. This remains a controversial issue. Both animal and vegetarian sources are listed in the chart below. If you have any doubts about whether or not your diet is providing you with enough B_{12}, consult your physician or a qualified nutritionist.

NATURAL FOOD SOURCES OF VITAMIN B_{12} (COBALAMIN)

Vegetarian*	Animal
Brewer's yeast (fortified)	**Lacto/Ovo**
Comfrey leaves	
Concord,grapes	Milk
Cereal (fortified)	Eggs
Kelp	Yogurt
Peanuts	Aged cheese
Raw wheat germ	Cottage cheese
Soy milk (fortified)	
Tempeh (a fermented soy	**Meat**
product with a meat-	
like texture)	Chicken
	Kidneys
	Liver
	Trout
	Tuna

*There is professional disagreement on whether or not you can get adequate amounts of B_{12} from vegetarian sources. Check with your physician or a qualified nutritionist.

CHOLINE

Choline works with inositol (discussed next) as part of lecithin, a substance found naturally in your body. Lecithin helps your body utilize the fat-soluble vitamins, A, D, E, and K. Some authorities do not recognize choline and inositol as vitamins, claiming there is not enough data to classify them that way. Others add them to the list that comprises the B complex. In addition to helping digest blood fats, choline

- Prevents fatty deposits in liver
- Minimizes cholesterol buildup in arteries
- Prevents gallstones
- Helps reduce high blood pressure

If you have a normal, healthy diet, your body can manufacture its own choline. Scientists are unsure of what the minimum daily requirements are; they estimate around 1000 milligrams. A long-term deficiency of choline can lead to high blood pressure, hardening of the arteries, and a buildup of fatty deposits in your liver.

FACTS ABOUT CHOLINE

Solubility: Water
Minimum Daily Requirement: None reported

Symptoms of Deficiency	Symptoms of Overdose	Things That Use Up the Vitamin Too Fast
Fat intolerance	Actual toxic dose unknown. (See remarks below and warning note on B vitamins at beginning of chapter.)	Alcohol
High blood pressure		Coffee
Cirrhosis of the liver		Sugar
Bleeding stomach ulcers		
Heart trouble		

Like vitamin B_1, choline is a water-soluble vitamin. Therefore the excess beyond what your body needs is excreted in the urine and does not normally build up. Scientists have not yet identified the toxic dose for choline. Remember our warning about the B vitamins: Always take them together in a balanced formula.

Choline can be found in several natural sources. As part of your effort to eliminate fat and reduce cholesterol, you should rely on vegetarian sources of choline.

NATURAL FOOD SOURCES OF CHOLINE

Vegetarian	Animal*
Brewer's yeast	**Lacto/Ovo**
Beans	
Green leafy vegetables	Egg yolks
Peanuts	
Soybeans	**Meat**
Lecithin	
Wheat germ	Fish
	Liver
	Kidneys

*Not recommended

INOSITOL

Inositol works with choline as part of lecithin, a substance found naturally in your body. Lecithin helps your body utilize the fat-soluble vitamins—A, D, E, and K. Inositol has been said to help prevent thinning of the hair and baldness. It helps to reduce blood cholesterol and to maintain a healthy heart muscle.

According to many researchers, your body can synthesize adequate amounts of inositol. Moreover, inositol occurs naturally in large amounts in many common foods. Scientists are not certain what the minimum daily requirements are, but estimates are generally the same as those for choline. A deficiency of inositol can lead to high blood cholesterol, eye problems, and constipation.

FACTS ABOUT INOSITOL

Solubility: Water
Minimum Daily Requirement: None reported

Symptoms of Deficiency	Symptoms of Overdose	Things That Use Up the Vitamin Too Fast
High cholesterol	Actual toxic dose unknown. (See remarks below and warning note at beginning of chapter.)	Alcohol
Constipation		Coffee
Eczema		
Eye problems		
Hair loss		

Like choline, inositol is a water-soluble vitamin. Therefore the excess beyond what your body needs is excreted in the urine and does not normally build up. The toxic dose for inositol has not yet been identified. Remember our warning about the B vitamins: Always take them together in a balanced formula.

Inositol can be found in several natural sources. As part of your program to eliminate fat and reduce cholesterol, you should rely on vegetarian sources wherever possible.

NATURAL FOOD SOURCES OF INOSITOL

Vegetarian	Animal*
Blackstrap molasses	**Lacto/Ovo**
Brewer's yeast	
Corn	Milk
Grapefruit	Yogurt
Lecithin	
Nuts	**Meat**
Oatmeal	
Oranges	Liver
Peanuts	Kidneys
Wheat germ	
Whole grains	
Vegetables	

*Not recommended

VITAMIN B$_x$: PABA (PARA AMINOBENZOIC ACID)

PABA is called the anti-sunburn vitamin because of its ability to protect against sunburn and skin cancer. It also helps with blood cell formation and promotes growth. PABA is often left out of multivitamin compounds because it makes sulfa drugs ineffective.

Your body can produce PABA in the intestines if enough friendly bacteria are present. Not much is known about PABA, but it has been used successfully in turning gray hair darker. It is commonly used as a sunscreen in suntan lotions and creams.

FACTS ABOUT VITAMIN B$_x$ (PABA)

Solubility: Water
Minimum Daily Requirement: Not stated

Symptoms of Deficiency	Symptoms of Overdose	Things That Use Up the Vitamin Too Fast
Eczema	Toxic dose is 10–100 mg. Dosages over 30 mg. require a prescription. Can cause heart, liver, and kidney damage. (See previous warning note.)	Alcohol
Depression		Coffee
Fatigue (extreme)		Sulfa drugs
Gray hair		Sugar
Anemia		
Infertility		
Reproductive disorders		
Headaches		
Irritability		
Constipation		
Digestion problems		

Always take B vitamins together in a balanced formula. PABA is *not* a harmless water-soluble vitamin. Some researchers report that high doses are toxic to the heart, kidneys, and liver.

PABA can be obtained from both plant and animal sources. As part of your effort to eliminate fat and reduce cholesterol, you should rely mainly on vegetarian sources.

NATURAL FOOD SOURCES OF VITAMIN B$_x$
(PABA: Para Aminobenzoic Acid)

Vegetarian	Animal*
Brewer's yeast	**Lacto/Ovo**
Molasses	Milk
Wheat germ	Egg yolks
Whole grains	Yogurt
	Meat
	Liver
	Kidneys

*Not recommended

VITAMIN C

Vitamin C promotes healing in all kinds of illness, protects against stress, and is a general detoxicant. It is extremely important to the functioning of your body's immune system. Vitamin C

- Helps your digestion
- Defends the body against toxins
- Helps you fight emotional stress
- Has been shown to prevent or reduce the symptoms of the common cold
- Is essential for healthy teeth, gums, and bones

Your body cannot synthesize vitamin C, so you must obtain it from the food you eat and/or supplements. The most basic function of vitamin C identified so far is its role in forming collagen, a body protein that makes up the tissue in your bones, teeth, skin, and muscles. Scurvy is due to a vitamin C deficiency.

FACTS ABOUT VITAMIN C (ASCORBIC ACID)

Solubility: Water
Minimum Daily Requirement: 30–70 mg.

Symptoms of Deficiency	Symptoms of Overdose	Things That Use Up the Vitamin Too Fast
Anemia	Toxic dose is 5,000 to 15,000 mg.	Antibiotics
Bleeding gums	Burning on urination	Aspirin
Breath shortness	Loose bowels	Cortisone
Bruises	Skin rashes	Tobacco
Low resistance to infection	Kidney stones	Stress
Muscle cramps		
Nose bleeds		
Poor digestion		
Scurvy		
Swollen joints		
Tooth decay		

Vitamin C is a water-soluble vitamin. Generally, vitamin C has been thought to be nontoxic and has been used in fairly large doses for the prevention of colds and to aid in healing infections. It is believed that the excess beyond what your body needs is excreted. Recent evidence suggests that it may cause kidney stones when taken in large dosages. We urge you to consult with your physician or nutritionist before taking large doses over an extended period of time.

NATURAL FOOD SOURCES OF VITAMIN C
(ASCORBIC ACID)

Fruits	Vegetables
Apples	Broccoli
Citrus fruits	Cabbage
Cantaloupe	Green pepper
Guavas	Potatoes
Papaya	Turnip greens
Rose hips	
Strawberries	
Tomatoes	

ANTISTRESS MINERALS

The body uses four minerals to ward off stress: calcium, potassium, magnesium, and zinc.

Warning: Do not take mineral supplements without the approval of your physician or qualified nutritionist.

CALCIUM

Calcium's major role is the formation and maintenance of bones; it is also a key factor in the contraction of muscles. Calcium is also essential to

- Blood clotting
- Maintaining a steady heartbeat
- Nerve transmission
- Healthy teeth

There is some evidence that calcium protects against the effects of radioactive strontium 90. Calcium is also essential for the effective metabolism of vitamins A, C, and D.

There is increasing evidence that a high-protein diet promotes calcium excretion. With age, the body is less able to absorb calcium, and many people are thought to be deficient in the mineral. Early signs are foot and leg cramps and insomnia.

FACTS ABOUT CALCIUM

Solubility: Acid
Minimum Daily Requirement: 800–1200 mg.

Symptoms of Deficiency	Symptoms of Overdose	Things That Use Up the Mineral Too Fast
Heart palpitations	Toxic dose not reported. May be side effects in some people.	Stress
Insomnia		No exercise
Muscle cramps		Too much saturated fat
Grogginess		
Nervousness		
Depression		
Porous bones		

Calcium should be taken along with magnesium; the usual ratio is two parts calcium to one part magnesium. Since we excrete 70 to 80 percent of our calcium intake, it is important for pregnant women and nursing mothers to have a sufficient calcium intake. About 90 percent of the calcium in your body is in the bones. According to many nutrition experts, the body replaces all its calcium every six years. If you do not get enough calcium from your food, it is withdrawn from the bones and teeth.

Remember, mineral supplements should be taken along with vitamin supplements in a balanced formula. As part of your effort to eliminate fat and reduce cholesterol, you should rely on vegetarian sources wherever possible.

NATURAL FOOD SOURCES OF CALCIUM

Vegetarian	Animal*
Almonds	**Lacto/Ovo**
Blackstrap molasses	
Broccoli	Milk
Brussels sprouts	Cheese
Cabbage	Yogurt
Carrots	Eggs
Dandelion greens	
Collards	**Fish**
Endive	
Grapefruit	Water-packed sardines

*Milk and milk products are the richest sources of calcium. Strict vegetarians may want to consider supplements.

POTASSIUM

Potassium might be called the anti-acid mineral because of its important role in maintaining the acid-alkaline balance of the blood. It also

- Helps your heart keep its proper rhythm
- Prevents low blood sugar
- Is essential for good muscle contraction
- Promotes hormone secretions
- May help prevent female disorders

Too much sugar can result in a potassium deficiency. Since potassium is essential to the metabolism of sugar and the formation of glycogen, a deficiency of potassium can result in low blood sugar.

FACTS ABOUT POTASSIUM

Solubility: Water
Minimum Daily Requirement: 2,000 to 2,500 mg.

Symptoms of Deficiency	Symptoms of Overdose	Things That Use Up the Mineral Too Fast
Acne	Toxic dose not reported	Stress
Insomnia		Alcohol
Muscle weakness		Coffee
Dry skin		Salt
Nervousness		Sugar
Excessive salt retention		Aspirin
Continuous thirst		Laxatives
Constipation		Diuretics
Muscle damage		Steroids
Extreme fatigue		
Low blood sugar		
Slow and irregular heartbeat		
Weak reflexes		
High blood pressure		

Your potassium intake should be about the same as your salt intake, but your exact potassium need may differ from other people's needs since it is related to the amount of salt you use. Potassium is an important part of the mineral base of your muscles and helps to make them flexible. Approximately 90 percent of your potassium intake is excreted in the urine.

As part of your effort to eliminate fat and reduce cholesterol, you should rely on vegetarian sources. If you are also using supplements, remember that mineral supplements should be taken along with vitamin supplements in a balanced formula.

NATURAL FOOD SOURCES OF POTASSIUM

Vegetarian	Animal*
Apricots	Lacto/Ovo
Bananas	
Blackstrap molasses	Milk
Dates	Yogurt
Green leafy vegetables	
Nuts	Meat/Fish
Oranges	Seafood
Peaches	
Peanuts	
Potatoes	
Raisins	
Sunflower seeds	
Whole grains	

*Not recommended

MAGNESIUM

Magnesium could be called the natural tranquilizer mineral because of its important role in the nervous system. Chemical fertilizers cut the amount of magnesium in food, and boiling or soaking food causes a greater loss. Magnesium

- Is essential for maintaining a healthy heart
- Helps the body retain calcium and potassium
- Helps your body regulate blood sugar and utilize fats and starches
- Contributes to the development of harder bones and teeth
- Helps build strong lung tissue
- Helps your body use vitamin E and B_1

Magnesium is an essential part of the process that makes the energy molecule ATP. It also helps your body maintain the desired acid-alkaline balance. Magnesium also helps your body use vitamin C and calcium. Since every cell in your body needs magnesium to function properly, a deficiency could lead to severe physical and/or mental problems. In addition, a lack of magnesium leads to calcium and potassium deficiencies, which in turn can cause kidney damage, kidney stones, and heart attack.

FACTS ABOUT MAGNESIUM

Solubility: Water
Minimum Daily Requirement: 350 mg. for males
300 mg. for females

Symptoms of Deficiency*	Symptoms of Overdose**	Things That Use Up the Mineral Too Fast
Rapid pulse	Toxic dose, 30,000 mg.	Alcohol
Insomnia		Excess calcium
Quick to anger		Too much saturated fat
Confusion		
Restlessness		Vomiting
Mental disorientation		Diarrhea
Tremors		
Seizures		
Premature wrinkles		
Kidney stones		
Muscle cramps		
Heart attack		

*Magnesium deficiency can cause loss of calcium and potassium, giving you their deficiency symptoms also.
**Since the intestines reject excesses of this mineral, it is highly unlikely that a person will experience a toxic overdose. However, people with kidney problems may do so. Symptoms of a toxic overdose may include extreme thirst, flushing of the skin, shallow breathing, and loss of reflexes.

Only about 30 to 40 percent of the magnesium you get from food is absorbed. The rest is excreted in both your urine and feces. Remember, mineral supplements should be taken along with vitamin supplements in a balanced formula. As part of your effort to eliminate fat and reduce cholesterol, you should rely on vegetarian sources.

NATURAL FOOD SOURCES OF MAGNESIUM

Vegetarian	Animal*
Alfalfa	**Meat/Fish**
Almonds	Seafood
Apples	
Bran	
Beet greens	
Brown rice	

Vegetarian	Animal*

Cashews
Dates
Figs
Green leafy vegetables
Honey
Lemons
Lima beans
Nuts
Oatmeal
Peanuts
Peaches
Raisins
Sesame seeds
Soybeans
Sunflower seeds
Whole grains

*Not recommended

ZINC

Zinc plays a key role in healing wounds and burns. In addition, zinc is required to form the insulin molecule and is therefore involved in carbohydrate and energy metabolism. Zinc also
- Is essential to bone formation and promotes good teeth
- Is necessary for proper blood clotting
- Helps maintain a proper heartbeat
- Is essential for muscle activity
- Protects against the effects of radioactive strontium 90
- Is essential for effective use of vitamins A, C, and D

A zinc deficiency can lead to reproductive organ problems, from delayed sexual maturity to an enlarged prostate to sterility. Early signs of zinc deficiency are white spots on fingernails and toenails.

FACTS ABOUT ZINC

Solubility: Acid
Minimum Daily Requirement: 15 mg.

Symptoms of Deficiency	Symptoms of Overdose	Things That Use Up the Mineral Too Fast
White spots on nails	Toxic dose not reported.	Alcohol
Sterility	Fever	Oral contraceptives
Delayed sexual maturity	Vomiting	Too much calcium
Fatigue	Diarrhea	

Symptoms of Deficiency	Symptoms of Overdose	Things That Use Up the Mineral Too Fast
Wounds heal slowly		
Burns heal slowly		
Enlarged prostate		
Hair loss		
Lowered sex drive		
Anorexia		
Diminished taste and smell		
Dandruff		
Low resistance to infection		

The zinc reserves in your body are not easily harnessed. Thus there is a need for an ongoing, regular intake of the mineral. This is particularly important during times of stress or periods of growth. Owing to the use of chemical fertilizers, there is less zinc in our soil and therefore in plants. But it is still available in various animal and plant sources. As part of your effort to eliminate fat and reduce cholesterol, you should rely on vegetarian sources. Remember, mineral supplements should be taken along with vitamin supplements in a balanced formula.

NATURAL FOOD SOURCES OF ZINC

Vegetarian	Animal*
Brewer's yeast	**Lacto/Ovo**
Green leafy vegetables	Milk
Mushrooms	Eggs
Onions	
Nuts	**Meat/Fish**
Soybeans	
Sunflower seeds	Liver
Wheat bran	Oysters
Wheat germ	Herring

*Not recommended

OTHER HIGH-ENERGY SUPPLEMENTS

In addition to the antistress vitamins and minerals we've discussed, there are several other supplements you may want to consider for your energy-building nutritional program. The more important ones include the fat-soluble vitamins A, D, and E and the minerals iron and selenium. All are important to good nutrition and offer significant protection against energy-draining environmental problems.

OTHER HIGH-ENERGY SUPPLEMENTS

Supplement	What It Does for You	Recommended Daily Allowance
Vitamin A	Helps resist infection Helps night vision Retards aging process Keeps testicles healthy Prevents eye diseases Nourishes skin and hair	4,800–6,000 IU*
Vitamin D	Promotes bone formation Prevents tooth decay Prevents gum disease Prevents rickets Keeps thyroid healthy	200–400 IU*
Vitamin E	Retards aging process Prevents scar-tissue formation Prevents blood clots Promotes healthy sex organs Promotes male potency	15 IU*
Iron	Prevents anemia Helps fight stress Promotes growth in children Builds up blood	10 mg. for infants 15 mg. for children 10 mg. for adult males 18 mg. for women of child-bearing age* 10 mg. for post- menopausal women
Selenium	Powerful antioxidant against air, water, food pollution Prevents red blood cell damage May slow down aging Reduces risk of cancer	Not established*

*Warning: Overdoses can be dangerous to your health. Do not take supplements without the approval of your physician

Chapter 12

Learn Which Are the Low-Energy Foods — and Avoid Them

The typical American today eats more and more food that has been sprayed, injected, dyed, chemically broken down and then reconstituted, bleached, frozen, and stored for months. To add insult to injury, this so-called food is loaded with salt and sugar—and then most of us sit down to a meal and add more. No wonder we have been described as overfed and undernourished. We call such foods low-energy food because they make you feel tired, because they drain your system of energy over a long period of time, and because they have an adverse effect on your immune system. Consuming low-energy foods may even lead to serious illness.

Take this quick quiz to test your knowledge of low-energy foods.

1. All-Bran cereal has less sugar than
   Shredded Wheat.   True False

2. Ketchup gets most of its calories from
   sweet, red ripe tomatoes.   True False

3. Medical science has found that sodium
   nitrate makes hot dogs, bacon, and bologna
   safe to eat.   True False

4. No one has ever died from eating foods containing sulfur dioxide or sodium bisulfite.   True False

5. Baking soda contains salt. Therefore you should use baking powder instead.   True False

The answers are all *false.*

1. All-Bran cereal gets about 29 percent of its calories from sugar; Shredded Wheat contains none. However, Shredded Wheat is packaged in paper impregnated with BHT, a preservative. Research shows a possible connection between cancer and BHT used with foods.

2. Ketchup gets 63 percent of its calories from refined sugar.

3. Sodium nitrate and sodium nitrite are used in hot dogs, bacon, ham, corned beef, smoked fish, and luncheon meats to help retard bacterial growth and to stabilize the red color. Unfortunately, these additives lead to the formation of cancer-causing chemicals called nitrosamines. Try a tofu hot dog instead!

4. Sulfur dioxide and sodium bisulfite are used as preservatives and to prevent discoloration in so-called fresh shrimp, dried fruit, and in some dried and frozen potatoes. They are also used to prevent bacterial growth in some wines. These additives have been found to cause severe allergic reactions and to destroy vitamin B_1 in your body. At least seven deaths have been attributed to them.

5. Baking soda contains about 821 milligrams (mg.) of sodium per teaspoon. Baking powder, while lower in sodium, still has a whopping 405 milligrams per teaspoon. There are low-sodium versions available that contain only 2 milligrams of sodium per teaspoon.

WHAT THIS CHAPTER CAN DO FOR YOU

You will discover:
- How our risk of developing some of our most serious diseases is linked to our intake of salt, sugar, caffeine, additives, preservatives, and refined foods
- How certain foods make us tired
- How to find alternative foods that taste wonderful
- What the newest research says about salt and sugar substitutes

THE "WHITE DEATH" FOODS

Salt, sugar, white flour, and white rice have been called "white death" foods. This is a rather melodramatic phrase, but it does highlight the concern we have about the quality of processed foods.

WHITE DEATH #1: SALT

Have you eaten at McDonald's or Burger King or Wendy's lately? Did you order the typical meal of a double cheeseburger, milk shake, French fries, and apple tart? Do you have any idea how much sodium you ate? Would you care to guess which food contained the most sodium? Believe it or not, the double cheeseburger is so far ahead in sodium content that it's not even a contest. The cheeseburger has over 825 milligrams of sodium. The French fries, with "only" 160 milligrams, have the lowest amount of sodium. The milk shake has over 200 milligrams and the apple pie has over 400 milligrams. In this one meal you managed to consume over 1600 milligrams of sodium—more than we recommend as your *total* daily intake—without even picking up the salt shaker. There are at least five good reasons why you need to limit your salt intake.

1. *Too much salt can kill you.* There is a direct link between salt consumption and hypertension. Hypertension, or high blood pressure, has been called the "silent killer" because in most cases there are no symptoms that announce its presence. Untreated hypertension can cause a sudden stroke or heart attack.

2. *Too much salt can make you tired.* There is a direct relationship between salt intake and tension levels. The more salt, the more tension. When you are under stress your immune system gets overworked. This drains your energy level.

3. *Too much salt can make you bloated.* Salt makes you thirsty, so you drink a lot of fluids. The salt then binds the fluids in your cells and tissues. You can put on several pounds of "water weight" after a typical Chinese restaurant meal, not to mention the extra inches around your abdomen and the swollen fingers and ankles that bloating causes.

4. *Too much salt can make you moody.* Sodium intake has also been found to be associated with the mood swings of women who suffer from premenstrual syndrome (PMS).

5. Too much salt can damage your kidneys. Fluid buildup puts excess pressure on all of your internal organs. They can take only so much pressure and still function properly. If one organ breaks down as a result of the pressure, others can be affected. Under these conditions your kidneys must work overtime. This can lead to or aggravate kidney problems. If your kidneys do not function efficiently, blood pressure can increase and possibly eventually damage eyesight and the brain.

"Where does all this salt come from?" you ask. "I don't use the shaker." But as we've seen, you can consume a lot of sodium even though you never use a salt shaker. Take Cynthia, for example. Though she is only thirty-three and slim, her blood pressure is high. Since she has a family history of hypertension and stroke, her doctor suggests she start taking antihypertensive medication.

"When I heard that I got scared," Cynthia said. "My father had a stroke as a result of high blood pressure. I had always thought of him as an active man, and it never occurred to me that he would ever stop being that way. My mother used to get angry with him for not following the doctor's advice, but Dad used to say he was sure God didn't want to see him too soon. Well, Dad was right. He didn't die, but he often says he wishes he had. After the stroke most of the right side of his body was paralyzed. I would cry every time after I visited him. So now you know why I'm scared. As soon as my doctor told me about my high blood pressure, I stopped using a salt shaker."

When we analyzed Cynthia's diet, however, she was shocked to discover how much sodium she was actually getting. We met in the early afternoon, so we analyzed only her breakfast and lunch.

Remember, this is just two meals' worth of sodium, and Cynthia never added salt to anything.

"HIDDEN" SODIUM

Meal	Approx. Mg. of Sodium
Breakfast	
1 cup Wheaties	355
½ cup milk	60
1 slice pumpernickel toast	182
1 serving butter	80

Lunch

1 serving condensed chicken noodle soup with water	1,107
2 slices beef bologna	440
1 slice American cheese	406
2 slices white bread	228
1 serving mayonnaise	78
TOTAL SODIUM	2,936 mg.

NEVER BE TIRED AGAIN RECOMMENDATIONS ON SALT

The Never Be Tired Again recommendation for a safe intake of sodium is to stay as close to 1,100 milligrams a day as possible. During our live-in program, participants get approximately 1,100 milligrams of sodium a day. No salt is added to the food during cooking, and there are no salt shakers on the table.

You can do the same in your own home. It's harder to control your sodium intake when you eat out, because chefs are notoriously heavy-handed with the salt shaker. Tell the waiter your doctor has put you on a low-salt diet (which is certainly true) and ask him to write *"No salt"* on your order. Don't order any dish that has a cheese or cream sauce—it will be heavily salted. And don't add salt once the food comes to your table.

Here are our Never Be Tired Again rules for salt:

- Don't add salt to food during cooking.
- Don't add salt to your food at the table.
- Read labels! Don't buy food that has had salt added to it. Salt comes under many different names, so when you are reading labels look for these words: *brine, bicarbonate of soda, monosodium glutamate* (MSG), *sodium alginate, sodium benzoate, sodium bicarbonate, sodium cyclamate, sodium hydroxide, sodium propionate, sodium sulfite.* Foods sold in health food stores shouldn't have any of those ingredients but may have other items with a high salt content. Avoid kelp, shoyu, soy sauce, and tamari.
- Eliminate or at least reduce the amount of salt called for in standard recipes if you bake, because you are also adding salt when you use baking powder or baking soda. This will not appreciably affect the taste.

If you buy food from the diabetic/low-sodium section in your supermarket, you are probably shocked by the difference in cost. Have you ever wondered why it costs more *not* to include an ingredient? *Nutrition Action Healthletter* recently quoted Dr. George Dunaif, a Campbell Soup Company executive, as saying, "To partly compensate for real and perceived loss in flavor with low and reduced sodium products, there is a necessity to add more ingredients, i.e., meat, vegetables, spices, and herbs. This adds substantially to the cost of these products." So now you know. These products cost a little more not because of what they leave out, but because of what they put in.

GET PRACTICAL ABOUT SALT

Are you a "salt addict?" Is life without salt barely worth living? You need to have a serious talk with the child inside you. At the mere mention of taking away salt that child gets angry. Admit it: You were feeling angry when you read the rules above. Now imagine this child inside you as a *real* child. Would you let him or her eat something that would ultimately do harm, even though the child got angry or begged and pleaded with you? Of course not; no rational adult would. You have to be the caring rational adult to your own inner child, and develop strategies to help reduce the amount of salt you eat. Here are some suggestions:

● *Cut down gradually.* Salt your food as you normally do, but instead of shaking the salt directly on your food, shake it into a cup. Then use only part of the amount of salt in the cup. Throw the rest away. If you're feeling quite brave, use only half of what's in the cup. Do that every time you salt your food for a week. It will help you get used to the taste of food with less salt. The next week, reduce the amount of salt a little more, and cut it down even more the third week. If you need to stay at any particular "salty" level for more than one week, do it. The important point is that you have made a commitment to cut down on your salt intake. How long it takes is less important (unless you have been diagnosed as hypertensive, and then it's critical to eliminate salt from your diet right away).

● *Have faith that you will learn to like food without salt.* It really is possible. We've done it ourselves, and so have many of our graduates. One man called us a few months after completing our program. "I knew you would get a kick out of this," he said. "I had a craving for my favorite dish, and it tasted too salty. I didn't enjoy it as much as I thought I would!"

SALT SUBSTITUTES

Spices are the perfect substitute for salt. You'll find ideas for their use in the excellent no-salt cookbooks on the market. There are also some excellent herbal mixtures available in health food stores and supermarkets. You can usually find them in the spice or diet sections. Put herbal shakers on the table and use them the way you would a salt shaker. Experiment a bit until you find the flavors you like best. Our favorites are put out by a family-run business called Potluck & Thyme, in Salem, New Hampshire. The owners, Ursula and Dick St. Louis, guarantee that their products contain "no salt, no sugar or corn-syrup solids, no fillers, no soy powders, no hydrolyzed vegetable protein, no kelp, no artificial colors or flavors, no preservatives and no MSG." They make three different versions: All Purpose Herbal Sprinkle, Seafood Sprinkle, and (our favorite) Gourmet Sprinkle. Each of the Potluck & Thyme products is available for about $3.00 plus shipping and handling. You can order all three in a wooden gift package that can go right on your table or kitchen counter. (For ordering information write: Potluck & Thyme, P.O. Box 1546, Salem NH 03079-1546.)

WHITE DEATH #2: SUGAR

Jimmy's parents aren't too concerned about what he eats for breakfast as long as he gets something in his stomach. Yesterday he had a Reese's Peanut Butter Cup and a Kellogg's Frosted Vanilla Pop Tart for breakfast. Cindy's parents insist she eat something nutritious for breakfast. She grudgingly consents to drink some commercially concocted fruit punch and eat a container of fruit-flavored yogurt. Who had the most sugar for breakfast, Jimmy or Cindy?

If you answered Cindy, you are alert to the latest nutritional information. If you thought Jimmy ate the most sugar, don't feel bad. You, along with millions of people, have been tricked by food manufacturers into believing the "healthy food" myths they have been promoting for years. Here is how the sugar content of the children's respective breakfasts breaks down:

Cindy has eaten just over one-quarter cup of pure sugar! If either of the youngsters has a soft drink during the day, it means another ten or eleven teaspoons of sugar. The list of sugar sources

Jimmy:

Food	Sugar Content
Reese's Peanut Butter Cup	5.3 teaspoons
Kellogg's Frosted Vanilla Pop-Tart	4.8 teaspoons
Jimmy's Total Sugar	10.1 teaspoons

Cindy:

Fruit punch (1 cup)	6.5 teaspoons
Fruit yogurt	6.0 teaspoons
Cindy's Total Sugar	12.5 teaspoons

goes on and on. It's in the cereal we eat for breakfast, the bread and soup we eat with lunch, the spaghetti sauce we have for dinner. Sugar contributes 53 percent of the carbohydrate in our diet. And what do we get for our 53 percent? Nothing but trouble!

IT'S NOT NICE TO FOOL MOTHER NATURE

When you eat carbohydrates in the form of whole grains, vegetables, and fruits, the pancreas releases insulin gradually into the bloodstream to deal with the glucose that is a product of carbohydrate metabolism. When you eat white sugar, your pancreas "freaks out." Why?

Because white sugar does not need to be processed in the same way as other carbohydrates and makes massive amounts of glucose available to the body immediately. Your pancreas senses this huge influx of sugar and panics. It's as if the pancreas were thinking, "Oh no! I must not have been paying attention. He must have eaten a huge meal when I wasn't looking. I'd better send along reinforcements so I can get this glucose processed immediately and normalize his blood sugar level!" Insulin surges into the bloodstream to round up the glucose, stores what it can in the liver as glycogen, and converts the rest into fat. The higher the insulin level, the more sugar is converted into fat. And the more fat you have . . . well, you know all about that from chapter 8.

Too much sugar makes you tired. Because your pancreas does such a good job, your blood sugar level falls rapidly. This puts you on a roller coaster ride: very high blood sugar just after eating the sugar, then very low blood sugar after the insulin does its work. Low blood sugar is associated with tiredness, irritability, fuzzy thinking, and headaches.

Too much sugar upsets your immune system. The symptoms of low blood sugar may make you crave another quick fix. So you have coffee and a doughnut or a candy bar. The roller coaster starts again, and the extremes of your blood sugar level play havoc with your immune system.

TOO MUCH SUGAR AND DIABETES

Diabetes occurs when the pancreas fails to produce enough insulin to deal with the glucose in the blood. But though we know *how* diabetes happens, we don't know *why* it happens. We do know, however, that there is a clear connection between sugar consumption and diabetes. For example, the United States has the second highest per capita consumption of sugar in the world; it also has the second highest incidence of diabetes. Scotland has the highest per capita consumption of sugar in the world, and—you guessed it—also has the highest incidence of diabetes.

The program we advocate contains all the nondrug elements medical research shows to be the most effective treatment for diabetes. Following the Never Be Tired Again program can significantly reduce and even eliminate the need for artificial insulin. One of our graduates in particular comes to mind. Rick wanted to lose weight and get his blood sugar under control, but at first resisted exercise and diet changes. After five days on our program, Rick's blood sugar was normal for the first time in seven years. What a difference it made in his attitude!

TOO MUCH SUGAR AND HEART DISEASE

Nobel prize–winner Linus Pauling claims that sugar is even more responsible for heart disease than fat is. The evidence that fat is the chief culprit is too overwhelming for us to give up our 20 percent fat rule. But we agree that sugar can be deadly. The high insulin levels it triggers stimulate the liver to make triglycerides, fatty substances that circulate in the bloodstream and have been implicated in heart disease. For reasons medical science does not yet know, high triglyceride levels are especially dangerous for women (cholesterol seems to hold the biggest danger for men). Excessive insulin also has been linked with decreases in HDL (high-density lipoprotein), the "good" cholesterol that carries fats out of the cells and to the liver for excretion.

TOO MUCH SUGAR AND TOOTH DECAY

Although sugary drinks are certainly bad for your teeth, they are not the only cause of tooth problems. Chewy candies, hard candies that you suck on for a while, and sweetened cereals all contribute to poor dental health. Interestingly, such junk food is not the only cause of tooth decay. Dried fruit can be just as much of a problem if it sticks to the teeth. So don't eat it without brushing your teeth afterwards.

TOO MUCH SUGAR AND OBESITY

Sugar has the same number of calories per gram as other carbohydrates—4, to be exact. But sugar is such a concentrated sweet that you can eat a lot more of it before you feel full. Sugar is stored as fat much more easily than complex carbohydrates, such as vegetables, beans, pasta.

Which do you think you could eat most easily: less than a quarter pound of chocolate fudge or three and a third large bananas? The fudge is worth 400 calories and its particular form of sugar (sucrose) will send your pancreas into a tailspin trying to get out enough insulin to deal with it. The bananas are worth about 280 calories if you can manage to eat three and a half big ones, and their form of sugar (fructose) will not set off the alarm that the sucrose will. You would have to eat four bananas to get the same amount of carbohydrate that you would get from less than a quarter pound of jelly beans. You have undoubtedly heard about the "empty calories" of sugar. When you compare the nutrients of the four bananas and the jelly beans, you find that the bananas have almost nine times the calcium, two and a half times the iron, almost fifteen hundred times the potassium, and forty times the ascorbic acid. The bananas contain 760 milligrams of vitamin A, while the jelly beans contain none.

As you eat more sugar, you have less room for more nutritious food. This means that your body must get all of its vitamins and minerals from increasingly smaller sources. Chances are that your body doesn't get all the vitamins and minerals it needs. So, contrary to what the advertisers tell you, sugar is *not* a good energy source.

TOO MUCH SUGAR AND PMS

Sugar, along with salt, has been linked with premenstrual syndrome (PMS). PMS symptoms include lower back pain, water retention, abdominal bloating, headaches, acne, insomnia, forgetfulness, agitation, mood swings, depression, cravings for sweets, and tension. If you experience some of the symptoms frequently, it might be wise to examine your sugar intake.

ALL SUGARS WERE NOT CREATED EQUAL

If you have a sweet tooth, don't panic. Although natural food sweeteners need to be used with discretion, some are better for you than others. The best food sweetener is one that is made primarily of maltose, a sugar that releases glucose into your bloodstream slowly and steadily. This means that you will not experience the quick jolt and quicker energy drain that refined white sugar gives. Maltose is about one-third as sweet as sugar.

THE BEST SOURCES OF MALTOSE-RICH SUGAR

- Rice syrup (made from rice) has a gentle sweetness. You can find it in most health food stores. Use it to sweeten salad dressings, baked goods, and beverages.
- Amasake (pronounced Ah-ma-*sah*-key) is a traditional Japanese rice sweetener with a delicate flavor. Use it in the same foods as rice syrup.
- Barley malt has a much stronger molasses-like taste, and is good in gingerbread or cookies.

The next most desirable type of sugar is fructose, or fruit sugar. The beginning stages of its metabolism require no insulin, therefore fructose does not cause a rapid rise in blood sugar or insulin. It is gentler on your blood sugar level than sucrose.

MOST COMMON SOURCES OF FRUCTOSE-RICH SUGAR

- Fruit concentrates. You can find a number of wonderful bottled fruit concentrates in flavors such as apple, black cherry, grape. They are made by well-known health food companies such as Hain and Bernard Jensen. You can substitute a fruit concentrate for the oil and sugar called for in baking recipes.

For example, if your recipe calls for ¼ cup of oil and ½ cup of sugar, use ½ cup of fruit concentrate instead. Mystic Lake Dairy, in Redmond, Washington, sells a delicious fruit concentrate blend of pineapples, peaches, and pears. It looks and tastes much like honey. (Call 206-868-2029 for information about a local distributor.)

- Crystalline fructose is a highly refined sweetener made by chemically splitting sucrose into its two component sugars—glucose and fructose. The fructose is then isolated and purified. While pure glucose has a glycemic index of 100, fructose has a low glycemic index of 20. (A food's glycemic index indicates how quickly and how high your blood glucose rises after you eat the food.) Fructose is sweeter than white sugar. Where sucrose has a sweetness rating of 100, fructose has a sweetness rating of 173. So you can use a great deal less of it to get the same amount of sweetness. It is still advisable, however, to think of fructose as "sugar" and to use it sparingly.

- Dried fruit is a great substitute for candy. Our favorites are dried pineapple rings and dried papaya. We cut them into pieces and keep them in a mason jar in the refrigerator. We can then take a small piece or two when the sugar craving strikes. Although its sugar is primarily fructose, dried fruit is a concentrated form of it. Don't think you can eat pieces of dried fruit with impunity, but if you have the discipline to eat small amounts, it is a real treat. Dried fruit's one major drawback is that it is often sprayed with sulfites, preservatives that can cause severe allergic reactions in sensitive individuals—they have been implicated in at least a dozen deaths. Sulfites are used for cosmetic purposes—to keep light-colored fruit from turning dark. Health food stores and some supermarkets carry sulfite-free fruit. Read the label carefully before buying.

The food industry has as many ways of including sugar in our food as it has for salt. There are also as many names for sugar as there are for salt. The following sugars raise the blood sugar level beyond the normal range:

SUGARS TO BE AVOIDED

- Honey is a controversial sweetener. Its sugar is half glucose and half fructose. When it is filtered, honey can be heated to

175 degrees or more. The high temperature affects the chemistry of the honey and increases the speed with which it is absorbed into the bloodstream. This raises the blood sugar level, causing basically the same reaction as white sugar does in your system.

- Maple syrup is basically sucrose and reacts like white sugar in your body.
- Molasses (blackstrap and sorghum) is also extremely high in sucrose and should be avoided or used most sparingly. Blackstrap molasses does contain B vitamins and iron, but there are other, healthier sources of these substances.
- High-fructose corn syrup is a liquid form of fructose. It is made by treating corn syrup with enzymes to change some of its starch to fructose. High-fructose corn syrup can contain up to 58 percent glucose, which makes it only minimally better than white sugar. The end result is a strain on your adrenal glands.
- Other sweeteners such as corn syrup, brown sugar, dextrose, invert sugar, raw sugar, and turbinado sugar are highly refined sweeteners that require insulin to be processed, and each will make your blood sugar level rise.

WHERE DOES ALL THAT SUGAR COME FROM?

According to the Center for Science in the Public Interest, here is a list of the major sources of sugar in your diet. No doubt you will recognize many of them.

- 100 percent of calories from sugar

Coca-cola	Kool-Aid
Pepsi-Cola	Certs
Mountain Dew	Jelly beans
Hawaiian Punch	Good & Plenty candy
Sprite	Most syrups
Tang	Popsicles

- 75 to 99 percent of calories from sugar

Nestea Iced Tea with sugar	Pine Brothers cough
Hi-C Grape	drops
Ginger ale	Cranberry sauce
Most chewing gums	Sherbets
Most jellies and jams	Most jellies and jams

- 50 to 74 percent of calories from sugar
  Honey Smacks cereal
  Apple Jacks cereal
  Ketchup
  Relish
  Chocolate toppings
  Sponge cakes
  Black Forest cake
  Cranberry juice cocktail
  Ovaltine Malt Flavor
  Dannon frozen yogurt, fruit
  Dannon frozen yogurt, vanilla
  Canned peaches, pineapple, pears (packed in syrup)
  Applesauce (sweetened)
  Crackerjacks
  Angel food cake
- 25 to 49 percent of calories from sugar

  All-Bran
  Frosted Mini-Wheats
  Sugar Frosted Flakes
  Froot Loops
  Quaker Instant Oatmeal
  Most cookies
  Most candy bars
  Applesauce cake
  Gingerbread
  Cupcakes
  Pound cake
  Yellow cake

  M&M's
  Chunky
  Liqueurs, brandy, cognac
  Ice cream sandwich
  Dannon low-fat yogurt with fruit
  Ice cream sundae
  Thick shakes
  Canned sweet potatoes
  Chocolate pudding
  Most pies

THE BITTER TRUTH ABOUT ARTIFICIAL SWEETENERS

Basically you can sum up the story on artificial sweeteners with the phrase "There's no free lunch." Here's why:

- *Artificial sweeteners can make you sick.*

When cyclamates first appeared on the scene nearly twenty years ago, everyone was ecstatic. Early research appeared to show they were harmless. But later research found cyclamates were linked to cancer and birth defects and the Food and Drug Administration banned them. Manufacturers are still lobbying to get them reinstated. Saccharin, which has been around for a century, has been linked to bladder cancer. Nevertheless, manufacturers got Congress to prevent its being banned; it still sells (with warning labels) despite a poor track record and bitter aftertaste! The verdict is still out on the newest artificial sweetener, aspartame. Some research indicates aspartame may cause behavioral problems and do brain damage to fetuses. The link between it and cancer is still being tested; safety questions linger. Our advice is: *Avoid all artificial ingredients.* Nobody really knows what the long-term risks are.

● *Artificial sweeteners will make you gain weight.*

Ironically, people use artificial sweeteners to cut down on calories so they can lose weight. Yet when researchers compared people who use artificial sweeteners to those who do not, the users were more likely to gain weight. No one knows why this happens. Michael Tordoff and Mark Friedman, psychologists from the Monell Chemical Senses Center in Philadelphia, think it is because a "sweet taste" stimulates the body to store more fats and carbohydrates. When this happens, your body naturally craves more food. MIT neuroscientist Richard Wurtman believes there is evidence that aspartame produces chemical changes in the brain that stimulate your appetite!

WHITE DEATH #3: REFINED GRAINS

Many years ago, before he went back to college, David drove a bread truck. In those days he really believed that enriched white bread would help him build a strong body. After all, his father was a baker and he accepted the superiority of white bread. Like David, many Americans believe "enriched" white bread is good for you. Isn't it? The answer is "No", on several counts.

Refined grains rob your body of essential nutrients. When wheat, rice, or any other grain is refined, two essential nutrients are removed: the bran (its protective casing) and the germ (its "heart"). Most of the nutrients are contained in the germ. For example, thirty-seven of the forty-four known nutrients that humans require are contained in whole wheat. Most or all of these essential nutrients are lost in processing. When the germ is removed you automatically lose two-thirds of the thiamine, a quarter of the riboflavin, and a quarter of the vitamin B_6 found in the whole grain.

There also is evidence that when you eat refined grains your body may rob *itself*, stealing essential vitamins and minerals from other sources in order to metabolize the refined product. This is a controversial idea at the moment, but it makes sense. Some of these vitamins and minerals, in particular the B vitamins, calcium, and magnesium, are antistress nutrients. If refined grains do rob your body of these protective elements, your immune system could be weakened.

Refined grains may increase your risk of cancer. In addition to removing the nutrient-packed germ, food processors also remove the bran. Bran is a nondigestible fiber that helps speed up the digestive process and is a key factor in protecting against colon cancer. Unless you get bran from some other source, your risk of colon cancer is higher than that of those whose diet includes whole grains.

OTHER FOOD ADDITIVES

There are several other potentially dangerous food additives to watch out for. Our advice, in general, is to avoid all additives whenever possible. The food business is a highly competitive, multibillion dollar business. It pours tons of money into research on marketing and shelf-life extension of its products. Since additives make it easier to sell the product, you can bet that they will be around as long as the public stands for them. Today millions of unsuspecting consumers are guinea pigs, unwittingly testing the long-term safety of numerous additives.

On the other hand, there are some additives that appear to be safe in terms of laboratory-verified side effects. Most of these are derived from vegetables (e.g., carrageenan from seaweed) or animals (e.g., casein from milk). You would think additives from plants and animals would be safe to eat. However, the effects of long-term use remain open to question in many cases. Thus corn syrup, which is used as a sweetener and thickener, is generally considered safe even though it promotes tooth decay. Unfortunately, it has no nutritive value—it's just empty calories. Indirectly, as an additive in a wide variety of not-so-nutritious foods, corn syrup may contribute to the breakdown of the immune system just as any other sugar will.

Don't be a guinea pig. This translates into the following rule: *If nature didn't make it or you can't pronounce it, don't eat it!*

The chart below lists some of the common additives found in supermarket foods and many restaurant dishes. The list is not meant to be comprehensive but to illustrate the problem of finding healthy foods.

SOME COMMON ADDITIVES TO AVOID

Additives	Problems and Risks
I. Food Colorings	
Blue Colorings Nos. 1 and 2	Cancer, brain tumors in mice
Red Colorings Nos. 2, 3, 40	Cancer, allergic reactions
Yellow Colorings Nos. 5, 40	Cancer, tumors, allergies
II. Artificial Flavorings	
There are hundreds. Most are used in junk foods.	Hyperactivity
III. Flavor Enhancers	
Monosodium glutamate (MSG)	Damage to brain cells of mice, severe allergic reactions in some people
Sodium chloride (Salt)	High blood pressure, bloating
IV. Preservatives	
The B's (BHT, BVO, BHA)	Cancer
The S's (Sulfur dioxide, sodium bisulfate, sodium nitrate, sodium nitrite)	Severe allergic reactions, cancer

CAFFEINE: AMERICA'S FAVORITE ADDICTION

Everyone is aware of the perils of tobacco and alcohol consumption. Nevertheless many people continue to smoke and drink. At least they have been warned about the dangers and it is, after all, their choice. But an addiction to caffeine has its own problems. Regular consumption of too much caffeine has been linked to birth defects, miscarriages, and fibrocystic breast disease. Too much caffeine can cause anxiety, nervousness, irritability, muscle twitching, nausea, and insomnia. The really sad fact is that our children become addicted to caffeine early in life, not from coffee and tea but from caffeine-laden soft drinks.

Is your child driving you crazy? Perhaps you should remove soft drinks from his or her diet. Not only will you get rid of the caffeine, you will also get rid of the eight to ten teaspoons of sugar in each drink. No wonder the kid is hyper—he or she is getting "high" on a double dose of sugar and caffeine!

A GOOD SOURCE OF UP-TO-DATE INFORMATION

If you want to learn more about salt, sugar, and other food additives, or simply want to keep up with the latest research on nutrition, consider joining The Center for Science in the Public Interest. This is a nonprofit organization that advocates improved health and environmental policies. As part of your membership you get a subscription to the Center's newsletter, *Nutrition Action Health Letter*. The Center also produces books, pamphlets, posters, and software on healthy living topics. (The address is: CSPI-ID, 1501 16th St., N.W., Washington, DC 20036.)

QUICK ENERGY CHARGE #5

Gourmet Garden of High-Energy Foods

Steps 1–5: See the instructions preceding Quick Energy Charge #1 in chapter 4.

Step 6: Energy programming

Breathing slowly and deeply, see the oxygen entering every cell in your body. See your tiredness and tension melting into the grass, leaving you relaxed and alert. With each breath, breathe in increased energy and breathe out tiredness and stress. See the energy come into your body as pure white light.

Now that your deepest self is tuned in and harmonizing in this relaxed but alert state, imagine yourself walking through a lush garden. Look at the beautiful, colorful, and bountiful rows of pure, natural fruits, vegetables, and grains. See yourself buying these wonderful, nutritious, energy-enhancing foods at your supermarket. Read the labels carefully. Notice that these foods contain no artificial ingredients. Imagine yourself taking this wonderful harvest home and preparing delicious, energy-promoting meals from them. Sense how your body and mind respond to your loving care, becoming more healthy, vigorous, youthful, and productive, more loving and compassionate than ever before.

Step 7: Reentry.

See the instructions preceding Quick Energy Charge #1 in chapter 4.

Chapter 13

Choose the High-Energy Foods and Never Be Tired Again

To survive, our bodies need carbohydrate, protein, and fat. Each serves a different function in maintaining a healthy, productive lifestyle. The energy report card below explains the differences among them in terms of your body's energy-production preferences. Please note, however, that we are grading them only on the basis of preferred ways to get energy. Each is important to your survival.

HIGH-ENERGY REPORT CARD

STRAIGHT "A"

Carbohydrates get the highest grade as a high-energy food. The fastest and most direct way to make high-energy molecules (adenosine triphosphate, or ATP) is with carbohydrates. Marilyn D. Schorin, R.D., of Rutgers Medical School, writing in *Nutrition in Clinical Care*, explains, ". . . the body shows a preference for energy derived from carbohydrate over that from fat. Even with plenty of fat still remaining after several hours of hard work, when the carbohydrate stores in the muscle are depleted, it is difficult to continue the activity." In fact, Schorin goes on to say, ". . . carbohydrate produces more energy during activity than fat does."

Glucose, the end product of carbohydrate metabolism, is the only energy source that can be used by the brain and the central nervous system. As we mentioned, it is also the preferred energy source for the muscles during activity, since carbohydrate produces more energy than fat does. For all of these pluses, we have to award carbohydrate straight A's in terms of energy production. There is no "B" energy source because carbohydrate is head and shoulders above the next source in line, which is fat.

A SOLID "C"

Fat is the body's second choice as a source of energy. We need a certain amount of fat, about 20 percent of total calories being the healthiest level. Fat not only stores energy but also protects the organs of the body from physical damage. To burn properly, fat needs the presence of carbohydrate. Without carbohydrate, the metabolism of excess fat produces ketones, which are poisons.

The body of course protects itself as long as it can. When it detects too many ketones in the kidneys, it will draw water from the cells to help flush the poisons out. In the process, however, cells are dehydrated and kidneys must work overtime. High ketone levels result in fuzzy thinking, a disruption in the sodium/potassium balance in the cells, tiredness, and high blood pressure. Because of these problems when fat is metabolized as energy, fat gets a solid "C" as a source of energy production.

THE NOT-SO-HOT "D"

Every grammar school student knows how important protein is. Your body uses protein to repair cells, build new ones, and as a building block in such vital compounds as hormones and enzymes. However, your body uses protein as a source of energy only as a last resort. One of the problems with using protein as an energy source is that a major by-product of protein metabolism is ammonia, which is quickly converted to urea (uric acid). Both uric acid and ammonia are poisons to your body.

If you follow the Never Be Tired Again recommendation of getting no more than 10 percent of your calories from animal protein, you can eliminate these toxic wastes with no problems. When your diet is high in protein, the uric acid and ammonia accumulate in your body, where they can cause gout, halitosis, fatigue, constipation, headaches, arthritis, kidney stones, and loss of calcium (which eventually results in osteoporosis). Moreover, a high-protein diet usually means you are eating fewer carbohydrates, which means you will have less energy. For all these reasons we grudgingly award protein merely a "D" for energy production.

The Never Be Tired Again program's top scorer for energy production, then, is carbohydrate. It is the most important source of energy because the body prefers to get its energy from carbohydrate.

HIGH-ENERGY FOODS FROM ANIMAL SOURCES

Any animal protein that gets less than 20 percent of its calories from fat is considered a high-energy food.

EXAMPLES OF HIGH-ENERGY FOODS FROM ANIMAL SOURCES

Food	Notes
Chicken and turkey	Look for poultry that is labeled as having no hormones or antibiotics added to it.
Fish	White fish has the lowest fat content. Dark fish, such as salmon and mackerel, have the highest concentrations of EPA (omega-3 fatty acids). These have been shown to decrease your risk of cardiovascular disease. Eat large saltwater fish, such as swordfish, tuna, and shark only occasionally. Because they are at the end of the food chain, they tend to have higher concentrations of toxins from polluted waters.
Shellfish	Shellfish are low in fat, as long as you don't fry them or smother them in butter.
Low-fat and nonfat dairy products	Although these are excellent sources of calcium, many people are sensitive to dairy products. They are very mucus-forming. If you think you have any sensitivity to dairy products, try a calcium supplement instead (see chapter 11). In any event, dairy products must be considered part of your protein allowance.

HIGH-ENERGY FOOD FROM PLANT SOURCES

Nature's vegetable garden is bountiful, with hundreds of foods to choose from. Be open to the possibility that you will discover new foods you will like as much and even more than foods you currently enjoy. David introduced Joely to collards and fordhook lima beans. Joely introduced David to artichokes and jicama (pronounced *hick*-a-ma), a hard, sweet vegetable that is delicious cut up raw in salads. Together we have experimented with bok choy (Chinese cabbage), Swiss chard (a green leafy vegetable that tastes like a buttery, mild-flavored spinach), fiddle head ferns, and squash blossoms. In addition to being delicious, vegetables offer some special healing properties:

SELECTED VEGETABLES THAT PROTECT YOU FROM DISEASE

Vegetables	Benefits
Carrots, spinach, collards, turnip greens, chard, tomatoes	These foods contain significant amounts of vitamin A, better known as beta-carotene. Beta-carotene protects against cancer of the larynx, lungs, and esophagus and has also been shown to heal and/or prevent ulcers. Robertson and colleagues, writing in the *American Journal of Clinical Nutrition*, reported on a study they conducted on the effects of raw carrot on serum lipids and colon function. Subjects were fed 200 grams of raw carrot every morning for three weeks. Their serum cholesterol decreased 11 percent and their bowels increased the elimination of bile acids and fats by 50 percent.
Brussels sprouts, broccoli, kale, cabbage, collards, cauliflower, kohlrabi	These are foods from the cabbage family, which research shows can protect against cancer of the stomach, bowels, colon, and lungs. In tests with animals they have been shown to be particularly effective against cancers produced by chemicals.
Garlic, onions	As part of a review of over 100 research studies on the medical effects of garlic and onions, Barry S. Kendler, Ph.D., of Manhattan College's Department of Biology, found that these foods do indeed protect against blood clotting. He also found evidence suggesting that garlic lowers cholesterol and triglycerides and is an effective treatment aid for hypertension. Fortunately, there are several garlic capsuled products on the market that work almost as well as fresh garlic but without the odor!
Legumes	Beans and peas, called legumes, are versatile foods. Beans make good soups, sandwich spreads, dips, and salad dressings, and serve as substitutes or extenders in all sorts of meatloaf and meat casserole dishes. In addition to "regular" beans—such as kidney beans, great northerns, white beans, red beans, black beans, fava beans, and the like—legumes include black-eyed peas, garbanzo beans (or chickpeas), green and red lentils, green and yellow split peas, and soybeans. Although most people think of peanuts as nuts, they actually are a type of pea in the legume family. Peanuts have a high fat content (approximately 70 percent of a peanut's calories come from fat), as do soybeans, which get 40 percent of their calories from fat. Legumes in general are an excellent source of fiber and help reduce cholesterol.

Fruits are a wonderful high-energy food. With the exception of olives and avocados, fruits are extremely low in fat. However, avocados are an excellent accent in a salad because their high-fat content (82 percent of an avocado's calories come from fat) is balanced against the low-fat content of the other vegetables. Fruits also have special healing qualities.

SELECTED FRUITS THAT PROTECT YOU FROM DISEASE

Fruits	Benefits
Apples, pears	Apples and pears are high in fiber and pectin. Pectin absorbs cholesterol, thus helping to clean it out of your system. "An apple a day . . . !"
Bananas	Bananas are one of the best desserts you can have. Although low in calories, they are one of the most complete foods. Low in salt and 99.8 percent fat free, they are excellent for low-sodium and low-fat diets. Bananas contain beta-carotene and vitamin C, both anticancer nutrients. They are also high in potassium, which is good for your blood sugar and your heart. Bananas are a good cure for traveler's diarrhea. They come in their own protective packaging and help replace potassium and other water-soluble minerals lost with diarrhea.
Apricots, cantaloupe, papaya, peaches, watermelon	These fruits are extremely high in vitamin A or beta carotene.
Olive oil	Olive oil, a monounsaturated fat, helps lower levels of "bad" cholesterol (LDL, or low-density lipoprotein) while raising the "good" cholesterol (HDL, or high-density lipoprotein). Olive oil protects against heart disease and blood clots.

Grains can be used in soups and salads, as side dishes, and as main courses in an almost infinite variety of ways. High in vitamins and minerals and low in fat, they are an excellent source of fiber. People tend to eat wheat, corn, and rice and forget about barley, buckwheat, millet, oats, rye, and triticale (a cross between wheat and rye). Quinoa (pronounced *keen*-wa) is a grain that comes from the Andes Mountain regions of South America; it was one of the staple foods of the ancient Incas. *Quinoa contains more protein than any other grain and contains all of the essential amino acids.* Quinoa takes just 15 minutes to cook and makes a nice change from rice. Look for it in your health food store. (See the Quinoa-Tomato Soup recipe, #11, in chapter 23.)

SELECTED GRAINS THAT PROTECT YOU AGAINST DISEASE

Grain	Benefits
Whole-grain brown rice	Whole-grain brown rice is an exceptionally nutritious food. It contains high-quality protein and complex carbohydrates. Brown rice protects against cancer and diabetes.
Oats, oat bran	Remember when your mother insisted oatmeal was good for you? She was right. Oats help control your cholesterol level and protect against heart disease. Oats have more nutrients than wheat or corn. Health food stores and some supermarkets now carry packaged whole-grain oat flour you can use in place of wheat flour. (See recipes #4, 5, and 6 for pancakes in chapter 23.) Sprinkle oat bran in soups and on your cereal. It doesn't have the harsh taste of wheat bran, and it will do more for your heart. If you follow our dietary guidelines you won't need wheat bran to provide fiber in your diet; you'll get plenty from the food you eat. And that's the best way to get fiber.

Complex carbohydrates are the preferred source of energy on the Never Be Tired Again program. They are also the preferred foods for preventing some major diseases:

THE CASE FOR EATING LESS MEAT

Research comparing vegetarians of all
varieties to meat eaters can be summarized as follows:

Disease	Findings
Cancer	Worldwide, the incidence of breast, colon, and prostate cancer among vegetarians is less than half that for meat eaters. Breast, colon, and prostate cancers are virtually nonexistent in underdeveloped countries where people live on a low-fat, low-protein, high-carbohydrate diet.

Heart disease and high blood pressure	Vegetarians have significantly lower levels of cholesterol. When a group of vegetarians were fed 8 ounces of meat a day for four weeks, their blood cholesterol rose 19 percent even though their weight did not increase.
	    Vegetarians have a significantly lower risk of heart disease.
	    Vegetarians have significantly lower blood pressure levels. One study of vegetarians found only 2 percent had high blood pressure, compared to 26 percent of the nonvegetarian control group.

Obesity, gout, diabetes, osteoporosis	Vegetarians on the average are thinner and weigh less than meat-eaters. A recent study showed only 15 percent of vegetarians are overweight, while 40 percent of average, meat-eating Americans are overweight. We would guess that most overweight vegetarians eat eggs and dairy products.

Disease	Findings
	The incidence of diabetes and gout is significantly lower among vegetarians. Vegetarians who eat no animal fat at all and who do not eat eggs or dairy products seldom suffer from adult-onset diabetes or obesity. They also show a considerably lower incidence of osteoporosis.

Although you certainly don't have to be a vegetarian to be healthy, the facts present a powerful case for cutting down on meat, eggs, dairy products, and fish. If you follow the Never Be Tired Again recommendations of not more than 10 percent animal protein, 20 percent fat, and the balance of your diet from complex carbohydrates, you will be able to maintain vibrant health and have incredible energy.

QUICK ENERGY CHARGE #6

Adventurous Eating

Steps 1–5
See the instructions preceding Quick Energy Charge #1 in chapter 4.

Step 6: Energy programming
Breathing slowly and deeply, see the oxygen entering every cell in your body. See your tiredness and tension melting into the grass, leaving you relaxed and alert. With each breath, breathe in increased energy and breathe out tiredness and stress. See the energy come into your body as pure white light.

Now that your deepest self is tuned in and harmonizing in this relaxed but alert state, imagine you are dining out at a fine restaurant. Seated across from you are the people you love most in the world. Look around the room and realize that every employee of the restaurant is there to serve your every need—fine food, pure food, delicious food, gourmet food, healthy food, all there for your asking.

Hear yourself ask for your favorite dishes prepared in new and bold ways. No oil. No butter. No cream. Just wonderfully spiced and flavored. Smell the aroma of the foods prepared for you. Sense the profound changes in the way your body now prefers gourmet food that is low in fat and protein and high in the energy you derive from carbohydrate. See yourself eating and immensely enjoying the taste, textures, and aromas of this wonderful repast—delighting in the knowledge that each bite is nourishing your body and creating a reservoir of boundless energy. Know that your adventures in gourmet, healthy eating have only just begun.

Step 7: Reentry. See the instructions preceding Quick Energy Charge #1 in chapter 4.

Part III

THREE INTERNAL ENERGY- PROGRAMMING TECHNIQUES

Chapter 14

Energy from Within

If you want to get all you can from this book, you must forget everything you were taught about the nature of reality. You have to get beyond the concept that matter is solid, that you are solid flesh. You have to get beyond the idea that your body has a fixed internal program that predetermines your physical condition. If you want to make exciting changes in your life, you need to understand and accept the idea that your mind and body are an energy system and that the laws of quantum physics apply to you.

Science took a dramatic leap out of the dark ages when it discovered that our bodies are made up of muscles, tissues, cells, blood, and bones. As scientific knowledge grew, we learned that our cells are molecules made up of atoms, and atoms in turn are composed of electrons, protons, and neutrons. Today we have instruments so sophisticated that we are able to study this world of subatomic energy. Not that anyone has ever actually seen an atom, mind you. Yet we know that atoms and atomic nuclei exist, because scientists have photographed and tracked the electromagnetic energy they emit.

Since you are made up of atoms, it's also true that at your most fundamental level of being, your body seethes with electromagnetic energy. It is fair to say your body *is* electromagnetic energy.

As we noted earlier, while the fact that our bodies are fundamentally energy systems is a new and exciting finding for Western science, it is old news to Eastern thinkers. Chinese medicine has known for centuries that the way to create healthy states of mind and body is to focus on balancing the energy fields that comprise our being. Since body and mind are part of the same energy system—your thoughts are a form of electromagnetic energy, too—both ancient thinkers and modern high-energy physics tell us that our thought waves can communicate at the subatomic level with the other forms of energy inside and outside our body.

Because the major messages of this book are so important, we want to reemphasize one of them: You can learn to develop this thought wave ability yourself. You don't need to be hooked up to a biofeedback machine to learn the techniques. You simply tap into your "energy consciousness."

Frank T., a recently appointed senior vice-president of a major financial services corporation, developed severe stomach pains the first month in his new position. They were subsequently diagnosed as symptoms of a bleeding ulcer. This was not the first time Frank had this problem. His bleeding ulcer syndrome only appeared when he was under stress—new job, new promotion, new house. We taught him a simple breathing exercise that he did faithfully for ten minutes twice a day. His ulcer symptoms disappeared within a week and haven't returned.

Sri Chinmoy's photograph appeared recently in *Vegetarian Times*. He was shown lifting 7,063 pounds of weights one inch off the ground with one hand. Before the lift he spent three hours in an altered state of consciousness, applying thought energy to the challenge. He had been lifting weights for only two years.

In his book *Beyond the Relaxation Reponse* (Times Books, New York, 1984), Dr. Herbert Benson reports on his studies of Tibetan monks. Dr. Benson verified scientifically, under controlled conditions, what Tibetans have known for centuries. At will, the subjects he studied were able to raise their outside body temperature by as much as 9 to 13 degrees in less than one hour of concentration. Contrary to the notions of Western medicine, the monks' internal body temperature stayed normal during these sessions!

Although being able to lift 7,000 pounds or change your body temperature at will may hold no special allure for you, there are benefits that may be of more interest.

QUICK ENERGY CHARGES: SELF-PROGRAMMING TO INCREASE YOUR ENERGY

Learning to use the special techniques we call "quick energy charges" has much more to offer you than just the ability to perform extraordinary physical feats. They are internal programming exercises we designed to ease you into a profoundly relaxed yet highly alert state of mind. The ability to reach this relaxed mental state can be your key to achieving inner peace and tranquility any time you want it, without having any other goal in mind.

REASONS TO USE QUICK ENERGY CHARGES

● *Your cholesterol is reduced.* Proper nutrition and exercise will make a dramatic impact on your cholesterol level. You can magnify these effects by using the quick energy charges described in the following chapters. We believe the reason our program gets such quick results in reducing cholesterol for so many of our clients is that we combine these techniques with our exercise-nutrition program.

● *Your risk of heart attack is decreased.* Quick energy charges bring about a profoundly relaxed state of mind. Studies show that your heart can actually slow down by as much as three beats a minute while you are in this relaxed state. This gives your heart a well-deserved rest. In addition, the incidence of irregular heartbeats is decreased. In combination with the effects of lowered cholesterol, slower heart rate explains why many who practice these techniques have lower risk levels for heart attacks.

● *Your blood pressure is lowered.* Many of those in our live-in program who had high blood pressure either got off their medication or reduced it in less than a week.

● *Your stress level is decreased.* At a biochemical level, the higher your blood lactate level, the greater your anxiety and tension. The techniques we discuss in the following chapters have decreased blood lactate levels nearly four times faster than simple passive resting. They also bring about a measurable increase in muscle relaxation.

● *Your energy level is increased.* The deep breathing involved in the quick energy charges increases the amount of oxygen in your blood. The relaxation component of the quick energy charges helps your muscles relax. When more oxygen-carrying blood flows through relaxed muscles rather than contracted muscles, more oxygen reaches all of the cells in your body. When cells have more oxygen they can manufacture more energy molecules (ATP). More energy is then available to you. Since the breathing and relaxation components of the quick energy charges also slow down your respiration and metabolism, your body can use the energy normally needed for those physiological functions for other purposes. The bottom line for you: more total energy.

● *Your ability to heal yourself is increased.* Variations of the approaches discussed in the next few chapters are being used in research centers around the world to heal cancer, control high blood pressure, and give people relief from chronic pain, asthma, bronchitis, back pain, chest pain, headaches, insomnia, and anxiety.

● *Your ability to control your weight is improved.* One theory on compulsive eating holds that our bodies simply don't get enough nutrients from the processed "plastic" food that most of us eat. And because our bodies are pretty smart, even when we aren't, they continue to cry out for more food in the hope that they will acquire the nutrients needed to maintain good health. The techniques of the quick energy charges have been shown to increase saliva production, which aids in the digestion and absorption of essential nutrients. This factor, coupled with internal programming statements designed to curb your appetite, can help you control your compulsive eating behaviors.

Note from Joely

When my mother read this section in its draft version, she penciled a note in the margin that read, "If I can accomplish all this just by doing the quick energy charges, why diet?" That question occurred to you, too, didn't it? Actually, it's a good question. It's true that you can accomplish miracles using only the techniques found in the quick energy charges. It's also true that changing your nutrition will do wonders for your health and energy. Exercise alone can make some people feel they have been given a new lease on life. We believe that human beings are too complex for any single approach ever to address fully. By combining approaches, you increase the effectiveness of each one. It is truly a case of the whole being greater than the sum of its parts.

● *Your memory and creativity are enhanced.* Several studies indicate that men and women who exercise their minds throughout their lives can actually increase their IQs! In a recent study, researchers found that the memories of sixty-two to eighty-three-year-olds were substantially improved when they combined the quick energy charge techniques with memory improvement training. Creativity is also enhanced when you regularly practice the techniques.

 • *Your performance and productivity are increased.* Numerous studies show that if you practice these techniques on a regular basis you can improve your performance on almost any task. The techniques in the next chapter, in particular, are used by business people to increase their negotiation skills, by sales people to improve their sales, and by Olympic athletes to enhance their chance of winning.

THE "RITUAL"

The methods described in the next three chapters all use what we call "programming statements" to tell your energy consciousness what you want to happen to your body, your health, and your energy level. You probably wondered why many of the statements are repeated in each quick energy charge. This repetition is for a good reason. It creates a familiar "ritual" that tells your conscious and subconsious mind to get ready for something important. The subconscious mind in particular learns well from ritual.

Chapter 15

High-Energy Daydreaming: Using Your Imagination to Banish Tiredness

Only in recent years has the idea of using the power of your imagination to achieve your goals or to improve your energy and health won credibility. In fact, many experts in the field of motivation who claimed success at harnessing this power were largely ignored by the general public; some were even labeled charlatans. But all that has changed. The use of guided imagery or imagery programming is now the subject of serious study in major universities and research centers. The knowledge gained from this research is already being applied—and is paying dividends—in the healing professions, athletic training, and the business world.

Consider the case of Bob, a sales manager who wanted to hire salespeople with a natural aptitude for selling. Bob asked a group of consultants to develop a formula he could use as a guide to hiring successful salespeople. The consultants began their work by comparing Bob's top salespeople with those whose sales record was below average. Surprisingly, the high sales group and the low sales group did not differ on any of the basic qualifications: Education was the same, age was the same, the years of training and experience were the same.

The consultants went back to the drawing board. They decided to conduct in-depth tape-recorded interviews of the most and least successful salespeople. After several weeks of interviewing, it still seemed there was no clear-cut answer to Bob's question.

As a last resort, the consultants decided to run a computer analysis of the transcripts. Lo and behold, they found the secret! The difference between the most and least successful salespeople was in their use of imagination! The top salespeople almost always used the technique of visualization, or "focused daydreaming," to meet important sales challenges. And they did so with greater intensity just before each critical sales call. They mentally visualized themselves getting their orders easily and smoothly. They saw their customers as completely satisfied with the deal. In stark contrast, less successful sales personnel did little or no daydreaming. In their interviews they talked about the sales challenges largely in terms of "problems." What they said to themselves about their ability to close a sale was defensive and self-protective rather than positive.

Bob set up a sales training program in which all salespeople were taught how to visualize positively as a regular part of their sales process. The result? Sales increased markedly, and Bob was soon promoted to vice-president of sales.

THOUGHTS COME FIRST

One of the newest and most exciting theories of high-energy physics offers an explanation of why imagery programming works. This new "superstring theory" maintains that all matter in the universe, at its most basic core, is composed of vibrating subatomic strings of energy. And, based on countless experiments, physicists have been forced to conclude that all forms of energy at the subatomic level are connected and able to communicate among themselves. In essence, energy communication at the subatomic level is what imagery programming is all about. The waves of energy your imagination creates communicate directly with the other forms of energy and matter in your body. They may also communicate with energy and matter outside of your body.

WHAT HARNESSING YOUR IMAGINATION CAN DO FOR YOU

Examples of the power of imagination are multiplying daily. Olympic training programs use a combination of relaxation and visualization techniques to enhance performance. In business, imagery helps executives prepare for important presentations, aids sales representatives to improve their sales performance, and enables professional negotiators to sharpen their skills. In psychology, a number of practitioners now use various forms of guided imagery to speed up the therapeutic process, to help people deal with career problems, manage weight control, and put clients in touch with their deepest emotions. In the field of physical healing, medical and psychological researchers around the world are experimenting with the use of imagery to strengthen the immune system and to encourage seriously ill patients to heal themselves.

Science is rapidly building the case that imagery techniques are not simply fantasy. For example, recent studies show that the simple act of *thinking* about jogging stimulates the muscle groups that are involved in jogging! We know the brain triggers the release of a chemical that causes muscle contraction. Even though we know this physical response occurs, we don't know why or how. From the viewpoint of superstring physics we can hypothesize that the energy in the thought waves communicates with the brain, stimulating it to produce the series of physical responses that result in a muscle contraction. Even so, we are only beginning to scratch the surface of the uses of high-energy daydreaming. David's experience with healing imagery is a good example both of the potential of the process and the closed-mindedness with which most medical practitioners still view the outcomes.

Now You See It, Now You Don't . . . David's Healing

When I was discharged from the army thirty-two years ago, the physician administering my discharge physical told me I had a weak abdominal wall. There was no doubt in his mind that as I got older I would get a hernia. I immediately put this thought out of my conscious mind, but I have often wondered if I unwittingly programmed my subconscious to produce the reality of a hernia in later years.

About twelve years ago I noticed a protrusion on the right side of my lateral abdominal wall about five inches below my navel. My family physician diagnosed it as a hernia. Several years later a surgeon who does numerous hernia operations each week diagnosed it as a rare form of hernia called a Spigelian hernia.

After several talks with my physician I decided to try healing the hernia myself rather than go in for surgery, even though I was told by several medical doctors and by my chiropractic physician that surgery was the only way to deal with it. In spite of their comments, I continued to visualize my abdominal wall as being sewn together with a strong Fiberglas patch; I imagined in my mind's eye that the wall would be stronger than ever. Within several months the pain went away; it has never returned. Thereafter I lived a normal physical life—running, swimming, doing yoga, and engaging in similar activities with no pain or distress. I must confess, however, that I did avoid heavy lifting.

However, the pouch of tissue that had formed around my hernia was growing larger. Even though I had no pain and did anything physical I wanted to, the pouch was an embarrassment. So after a long period of contemplation I opted for surgery. When the surgeon opened me up, he found a healed abdominal wall under the pouch. At the postoperative examination he also discovered that all of my abdominal walls were normal. Needless to say, none of the physicians would accept that I had healed my own hernia through imagery. Instead, they decided that all the physicians who had originally diagnosed it as a hernia were wrong!

IMAGERY PROGRAMMING

Do you remember your first love? You probably went through a period in the relationship where you did a lot of daydreaming about what it would be like to be married to that wonderful person. The difference between the daydreaming of your youthful ardor and the kind of imagery we are talking about is that you do it in a focused and purposeful fashion under more controlled conditions. There are three types of imagery programming you can use:

TYPE I: THE LASER BEAM APPROACH

With this approach you aim your thought waves at a specific target or goal. The targeted change can be an area of your body you want healed, a job promotion you desire, a relationship that you want to repair, and so on. When you program with the laser beam approach, you create a highly specific image of your goal and project it on your imagination "screen" by focusing on it to the exclusion of all other thoughts. This is the type of imagery David used to heal his hernia. Using laser beam imagery is very straightforward. Simply build a concrete picture of what you want to happen.

Here are two examples of using the laser beam imagery for physical healing:

- When David wanted to heal his hernia, he saw the gap in his abdominal wall being closed with a Fiberglas patch so that the wall was stronger than ever.

- If you want to lower your cholesterol level you might envision little "helpers" hosing down the walls of your arteries and washing away the accumulated plaque. Then you might "see" trucks with HDL written on the side loading up shovelfuls of cholesterol and carrying them to the liver to be excreted. (HDL is high-density lipoprotein. It is called "good cholesterol" because it carries cholesterol out of the cells and to the liver for excretion.) Although this image is a representation of what actually happens on the physical level, it doesn't matter what kind of image you use as long as you make it specific and positive.

TYPE II: THE INTERNAL THEATER

Each of us has a "guide" inside us that is always available. Depending on your background, you may call this guide "Spirit," "higher consciousness," or "guardian angel." You may think of this guide as your higher self or perhaps as the embodiment of an actual person whom you would like to have as your teacher. In this second type of imagery programming, which we call the internal theater, the focus is on using your personal guide (or guides) to help you gain insight into your problem. You are the audience and your guide(s) are the main actors.

The scenes of the play unfold this way:

1. You follow the relaxation sequence of the quick energy charges and in your mind you go to a particular setting or sanctuary.
2. When you get there you ask your guide or guides to join you.
3. When they arrive you pose a specific question and ask for their help. For example, you could ask, "Why am I having such difficulty sticking with an exercise program?"
4. You then wait for the answer(s) to come to you, either in images, words, or thoughts on your imagination screen.
5. Take whatever answer comes without judging it, and

continue to ask the question until there are no more answers. You will be amazed at the answers that come up.

TYPE III: THOUGHT SCAN

Have you ever been on a long car trip and used the station scan button on your car radio? It will pick up the strongest station in the area and then stop scanning. You can listen to that particular station or push the button again and it will continue to scan to the next strongest station. Similarly, thought scan imagery involves scanning your mind for specific answers to a specific problem. Thought scan works best if you are relaxed. During a thought scan, you do not actively choose the images. You allow them to appear on your imagination screen for your consideration. You allow your own subconscious to communicate with your conscious mind.

One of the basic challenges in imagery programming is preventing your emotional hangups from blocking your positive programming. Negative thoughts, especially unconscious ones, create interference or static in the superstring communication.

Not all negaive thoughts are unconscious. Some are right up front. Suppose, for example, you want to run in the local ten-kilometer race. You sign up, and then what happens? All of a sudden you begin to hear a little voice inside of you saying over and over again, "Remember your bad ankle. You'll never make it. You're not a kid anymore. What's wrong with you?" You've experienced this kind of negative static before, we're sure. All you have to do to push it away is to say to yourself, "Isn't it interesting that part of me feels that way? But I'm still going to enter the race. And I'm going to finish. And my ankle is getting stronger and stronger every day." It's really easy to get rid of this kind of static because it is conscious thought; it is right there in the forefront of your mind. The trick is to discover the negative thoughts that you have stored in your unconscious.

The thought scan technique is an excellent way to help you unearth your hidden negative emotional thoughts and to stop them from clogging up your energy communication lines. Once you know what they are, you can deprogram yourself by substituting positive thoughts. Next time you are stuck on a business or personal problem, try the thought scan to find out why you are blocking your own creative energy. It's one of the best ways we know to get the "garbage" out of your system.

THE ELEVEN SECRETS OF IMAGERY
PROGRAMMING

If you were a naturally talented runner, would you assume you could become an Olympic champion without practice? Of course not! If you wanted to win the gold you would have to practice and train every day. Imagery programming is much the same. The ability to use one's imagination is a natural human attribute. However, harnessing the power of imagination to change or improve your energy level requires regular practice. The eleven secrets we're going to share with you will help your practice go more smoothly.

SECRET #1: TAKE ENOUGH TIME

Most people don't take the time to truly relax. Instead, they pop a tranquilizer or lose themselves in watching television. Taking medication may be appropriate at times. Idling away an hour or so with television can be fun. But neither is a substitute for focused relaxation. Don't cheat yourself by rushing through the relaxation portion of the quick energy charges. The more relaxed you become, the more effective your imagery programming.

SECRET #2: USE YOUR BRAIN POWER

Your brain contains millions of cells. Each one emits a measurable electrical charge called a brain wave. We have four different frequencies of brain waves, each associated with a different state of consciousness. Each has a specific shape that identifies it on the electroencephalograph.

- *Delta waves* are the slowest brain wave frequencies and are linked with very deep sleep.
- *Beta waves* most often appear when you are alert and concentrating.
- *Theta waves* occur just before you fall asleep; they also have been recorded at the exact time when sleep-experiment subjects report having key insights or inspirations.
- *Alpha brain waves* are associated with deep relaxation.

Science has not been able to determine whether alpha waves cause deep relaxation, or whether deep relaxation increases the production of alpha waves. Nevertheless, if you follow the relaxation component of the quick energy charges, you will not only be more relaxed, you will also increase your alpha/theta waves. It is not surprising that people who meditate on a regular basis report that they have more creative insights, feel more in control of their lives, and are less stressed and more productive.

SECRET #3: COMMUNICATE WITH YOUR ENERGY CONSCIOUSNESS

Let your body know how you want it to behave. Program it for positive results. You probably have conversations with yourself all day long without actually being aware of them. The things you say to yourself during those conversations ("self-statements," some psychologists call them) are extremely important. They have a tremendous impact on your life. Think about how many times you say nasty and negative things to yourself—things like "You dummy! How could you do such a stupid thing" or "I'm so clumsy!" or "I'm such a fat slob! I look a mess."

Each of us has a little child inside of us. If you want that child to grow strong and self-confident, you must say positive and encouraging things to it. What do you think would happen if you said all those negative things to a real child?

An Imaginary Case Study

Imagine that you have identical twin children. Because they are identical, everything about them is the same except for the fact that you always speak positively to one and negatively to the other. When twin #1 builds a house with blocks you say, "That's absolutely wonderful. You're such a smart person. I'll bet you can do anything you set out to do." When twin #2 builds the same house you say, "That's a pretty dumb-looking house. Why didn't you leave space for a door? How do you expect people to get in and out, stupid? You're not a very good block builder. Why don't you try coloring? But make sure you're not messy like you usually are."

You really couldn't expect the twins to grow up with the same approach to life. You've beaten poor little twin #2 into the ground. Yet that is precisely what you are doing to the small child inside yourself when you constantly say negative things to yourself. Start listening closely to your self-statements. Write down every negative remark. You will be shocked, but the shock should help you be more aware of how often you do this. To break yourself of the habit, examine every negative self-statement you make. Then substitute a more positive one. If you said, "How could I be so stupid as to make such a careless mistake?", try congratulating yourself for catching the error. Then say something like "I'll fix it right away and I'll be more careful next time. I'm really a careful person."

The same principle that applies to the child part of your psyche applies to your body. How often do you get up in the morning not feeling quite chipper and face the choice of how you want your body to feel for the rest of the day? If you have something important to do or something you especially want to do, you probably tell yourself this is no time to be sick, and then go about your affairs. Your sick feelings more than likely disappear during the day and you never think about them again. On the other hand, if you don't really want to do what's on the day's schedule, you'll probably decide you feel poorly and go back to bed. By the end of the day you probably feel downright sick. What makes the difference in how you ultimately feel on those two occasions is the way you communiate with your energy consciousness—the message you send to your cells. Pay particular attention to the sections in the quick energy charges where you are asked to focus on sensing and harmonizing your energy vibrations. This is where your most powerful imagery programming begins.

SECRET #4: USE THE PRESENT TENSE WHEN PROGRAMMING

It is important that your inner message be specific, clear, and in the present tense. Your energy consciousness can't translate future tense into action. Instead of saying "I will be healed," say "I am healed" or "I am healing."

SECRET #5: HARNESS THE POWER OF WINNING STATEMENTS

Dr. Norman Vincent Peale said it. Dr. Robert Schuller said it. Dr. Denis Waitley said it. They said, "Think positively." They will also tell you that they did it themselves. These best-selling authors have sold millions of books on how to be successful! Based on the testimonials they have received, many of their readers followed their advice and became successful, too.

All these folks have been preaching and/or following a law that has been with us for millennia. The Bible version reads, "As ye sow, so shall ye reap." In other words, you get back what you put out there. If you say you "can't," believe us, you can't. Psychologists call it the self-fulfilling prophecy. You remember the story of the little train that learned to say "I think I can, I know I can" and made it up the steep grade. The message of the power of positive statements was right there for you in your nursery school class. Did you pay attention?

Too many people send pessimistic messages to themselves and the universe. In some cases these negative energy signals continue throughout a person's lifetime, creating waves of illness, of unhappiness. Consider the evidence of a recent study conducted at a major university:

Your Thoughts May Be Dangerous to Your Health

Scientists Christopher Peterson, of the University of Michigan; Martin Seligman, of the University of Pennsylvania; and George Vaillant, of Dartmouth University, found they could predict the physical health of people based on statements the subjects had made nearly forty years earlier. The researchers had access to questionnaires completed in 1946 asking a group of soldiers about difficult experiences in World War II. The men were classified as optimists if they considered the negative event to be a function of the times, of passing duration, and not reflective of their life in general. In contrast, pessimistic men considered the negative event to be part of a larger negative life picture—"That's the story of my life." Forty years later, researchers correlated the verbal statements made during the war to the veterans' current health histories and lifestyles. They found veterans who optimistically interpreted wartime events stayed healthy and robust throughout their lives. Those with a pessimistic view of the events had long histories of chronic illness. What kind of statements do you make about your life events? They can be as optimistic and positive as you choose to make them.

SECRET #6: GIVE BACK TO THE SYSTEM

An old technique for tuning your energy consciousness into the larger system is the idea of casting your bread upon the waters— giving freely to others with no expectation of return. Usually you get back more than you give. Many people today spend much of their lives seeking to acquire material possessions. They work long hours to earn money to buy the latest gadget they see advertised. Then they grow frustrated because despite their efforts they fail to get the things they most want.

That happens because these men and women do not have a basic understanding of how the universal energy system works. If you think of the system as an underground ocean of pure water, the only way you are going to get that water up to your level is to "prime the pump." The more you prime the pump, the more water you are going to get. The remarkable thing is that the source of water is infinite!

About five years ago we had our eyes opened to how this works:

Why the Rich Stay Rich

At one time we owned a consulting firm that did research and training for businesses. One of our assignments was to find out why some stockbrokers were consistently successful and others were not. We were given access to the top one hundred brokerage firms in the country. We interviewed the top producers in these firms and compared their answers to those of the typical stockbroker. Our questions involved work habits, lifestyles, and personal backgrounds.

After a complex statistical analysis of the replies, we found twelve characteristics in which the top producers differed significantly from the others. These ranged from taking responsibility for their successes and failures to being able to laugh at themselves to taking responsibility for their health. (Yes, those who were the most successful also tended to be the ones who exercised and watched what they ate.)

Another important characteristic of this top group is that they had a "giving" attitude. This group of top producers included some of the most financially successful people in America. And, yes, they all had a long history of "giving back" to the system. Their giving was not just in the form of money; they devoted much of their time and labor to worthy causes. They also served as mentors to young people on their way up. They all claimed that they received more from what they "gave" than the people and causes they gave to.

SECRET #7: DON'T EVER GIVE UP

No one ever achieved anything by quitting. One of our former business clients, at the time president of a prestigious financial institution, always talked about the 90-10 percent rule of management. He said most people break their necks to get a job done, but usually only up to a critical point. At about the 90 percent level of task completion, most people lose their steam and motivation.

That's when our client would bring in a new management team to make that remaining 10 percent of the job someone else's 90 percent challenge!

When you think about it, our client's diagnosis of the human condition is true. Most people give up. And because they give up, they lead lives of quiet desperation. Whether it is in business, academia, or in the professions, perseverance is the difference between the few who fulfill their dreams and the many who do not. There's a quote attributed to Calvin Coolidge that says it all:

Press On

Nothing in the world can take the place of persistence. Talent will not; nothing is more common than unsuccessful men with talent. Genius will not; unrewarded genius is almost a proverb. Education alone will not; the world is full of educated derelicts. Persistence and determination alone are omnipotent.

SECRET #8: ABUNDANCE IS YOUR BIRTHRIGHT

Abundant energy, abundant health, abundant love, abundant material goods, and abundant food, clothing, and shelter are possible for everyone. The universe is an infinite network of unrealized energy.

Start today. Let go of your belief in the Western ethic that success depends on *hard* work and *sacrifice*. Let go of the Eastern idea that all life is suffering. You have the power to create your own abundant reality without diminishing anyone else's life. The "way" is to participate fully in your own life. Take charge. Choose to do the things you really want to do to earn your living. It's amazing how the universe will reward you if you choose to do what you were sent here to do. And only you know what that is.

SECRET #9: YOU DON'T HAVE TO GET IT RIGHT

Even though we have made suggestions about how to do imagery programming and the quick energy charges, there is no single "correct" way to do them. Every client we have worked with has his or her own way of doing them. Any way that works for you is right.

SECRET #10: ACCEPT YOUR RANDOM THOUGHTS!

As we mentioned earlier, it is perfectly normal to have thoughts enter your head that are not part of your imagery programming plan. The way to deal with these random thoughts is to accept their interference passively. Even if the thoughts are negative, don't buy into them. Stay passive. Let them pass through your mind like fluffy white clouds. Then get on with your positive imagery programming.

SECRET #11: GIVE YOURSELF A BREAK

You will wander and stray from the new path you have chosen. So what? Notice when it happens. Say, "Well, that's interesting." And go back to being active in your life change process.

SAMPLE IMAGERY EXERCISES

Each time you repeat the relaxation section of the quick energy charges, your level of relaxation and your ability to self-program are deepened and intensified. We have included quick energy charges for healing and weight loss in this chapter. Use these as a model to create your own versions, with programming statements geared specifically to *your* personal situation and needs.

QUICK ENERGY CHARGE #7

A Healing Imagery

Steps 1–5: See the instructions preceding Quick Energy Charge #1 in chapter 4.

Step 6: Energy programming
Breathing slowly and deeply, see the oxygen entering every cell in your body. See your tiredness and tension melting into the grass, leaving you relaxed and alert. With each breath, breathe in increased energy and breathe out tiredness and stress. See the energy come into your body as pure white light.

Now that your deepest self is tuned in and harmonizing in this relaxed but alert state, say to every cell, to every energy string in your body, "I have chosen to be healed. I am healing now. With each passing day I am getting more and more healthy." Shine your mind's flashlight on every cell in your body. See your body manufacturing an endless stream of high-energy white cells that destroy with ease all the harmful bacteria and viruses in your body. See your body constantly being rejuvenated, cell by cell, as you breathe in healing oxygen with each breath.

Note: At this point you can use images for specific body parts. For example, if you have a twisted ankle, you can shine your mind's flashlight on the ankle. See it getting stronger, more relaxed, see the swelling going down as the ankle heals. See an image of yourself walking free of pain, with ease, completely healed.

Look in an imaginary mirror and see yourself growing younger, stronger, and more creative with each passing day. Follow that thought deep into the mirror of your mind and beyond, all the way to infinity, constantly creating a younger, stronger, healthier, more self-confident You.

Now, enhance the program by clearing your mind of all other thoughts except the picture of the younger, stronger, more creative You in the miror. Notice how comfortable you feel with this image of yourself. Let the fundamental energy vibrations that are you sense the permanence of this healing decision that you have made. Feel your energy vibrations communicating this new knowledge to the universal network of vibrating energy strings, and know that it is understood.

Step 7: Reentry. See the instructions preceding Quick Energy Charge #1 in chapter 4.

QUICK ENERGY CHARGE #8

Weight Loss Imagery

Steps 1–5: See the instructions preceding Quick Energy Charge #1 in chapter 4.

Step 6: Energy programming

Breathing slowly and deeply, see the oxygen entering every cell in your body. See your tiredness and tension melting into the grass, leaving you relaxed and alert. With each breath, breathe in increased energy and breathe out tiredness and stress. See the energy come into your body as pure white light.

Now that your deepest self is tuned in and harmonizing in this relaxed but alert state, say to every cell, to every energy string in your body, "I have chosen to enjoy food that is healthy for me. I eat three satisfying meals a day and healthy snacks between meals when I want. When I crave food that does not nourish or heal, I have a healthy substitute ready that I enjoy. With each passing day, I am more toned and fit as my body assumes its normal, healthy weight level. Each day I get younger and healthier."

Shine your mind's flashlight on every cell in your body. See your body manufacturing an endless stream of high-energy cells that nourish and heal you. See your body constantly being rejuvenated, cell by cell, as you inhale healing oxygen with each breath.

Note: At this point you can use images for the specific body parts you want to be toned. For example, you might see an image of your waist going from a size 36 to a size 32 as you eat healthier foods. Actually see yourself going into a store and buying new clothes because your waist has shrunk four inches.

Look in the imaginary mirror of your mind and see yourself getting younger, stronger, and more toned with each passing day. Follow that thought deep into the mirror of your mind and beyond, all the way to infinity, constantly creating a younger, stronger, more healthy, more self-confident You.

Now enhance the program by clearing your mind of all other thoughts except the picture of the younger, stronger, more creative You in the mirror. Notice how comfortable you feel with this image of yourself. Let the fundamental energy vibrations that are you sense the permanence of your weight-loss commitment. Feel your energy vibrations communicating this new knowledge to the universal network of vibrating energy strings. And know that it is understood.

Step 7: Re-entry. See the instructions preceding Quick Energy Charge #1 in chapter 4.

Chapter 16

New Ways You Can Use Old Rituals to Conquer Tiredness

Lorraine B. rides the commuter train from Scarsdale, in suburban Westchester County, to Manhattan's Grand Central Station every morning. Unlike the horde of other corporate executives and Wall Street whiz kids who travel this route daily, Lorraine doesn't read the *New York Times* or the *Wall Street Journal* on the morning ride. Instead, she finds a seat, closes her eyes and begins to breathe in and out slowly. She counts each breath as she exhales. When she reaches the count of eight, she repeats the count again from one. If she is interrupted, she simply begins again. Lorraine continues this procedure for the entire forty-five-minute trip. When she arrives at Grand Central she feels energized and amazingly calm at the same time.

Jim S. takes a different kind of coffee break from most of Chicago's high-pressured advertising executives. He takes what he calls a blood pressure pill break. Only Jim doesn't take medication. Instead, he has his secretary hold all calls and visitors from ten to ten-fifteen every morning. He draws the blinds in his office, sits straight in his chair, closes his eyes, and begins breathing in and out slowly. As he exhales he says to himself, "One." He repeats this routine for fifteen minutes. He no longer needs the high blood pressure medication that he had been taking for three years.

Mary J. works evenings as a *maitre d'* in one of San Francisco's finest dining establishments. The restaurant is always packed; it sometimes takes two weeks to get a reservation. When Mary gets home at three in the morning she falls into bed, physically exhausted from the pressure of her job. Every morning Mary rises at eleven, spends thirty minutes exercising on her treadmill, and takes a leisurely shower. Then, dressed in a loose white robe, she goes to her "quiet room." There, sitting cross-legged in front of a low stool, she lights the candle that rests atop the stool. Mary closes her eyes and takes three long, slow, deep breaths. Then she opens her eyes and stares at the candle's flame. Each time her mind wanders she lets the thoughts pass, continuing to stare at the flame. Sometimes she closes her eyes and tries to keep the image of the candle and flame in her mind. When the image fades she opens her eyes and repeats the process. This routine lasts about twenty minutes. Since Mary began observing this daily ritual, her spastic colon has healed, and the blinding headaches that once plagued her are a thing of the past.

Mary, Jim, and Lorraine have two things in common:

- All three have high pressure jobs.
- All three have discovered a powerful way to reduce their level of anxiety and stress without the use of drugs.

The routines that Mary, Jim, and Lorraine use are simply variations on meditation techniques that have been developed through the ages in such places as India, China, Tibet, Japan, and Christian monasteries. In the past twenty years or so, these techniques have been refined by psychological research teams at major universities. We have combined all these methods under the label of "Total Concentration." Like imagery programming, the scientifically established benefits of practicing Total Concentration are amazing.

TOTAL CONCENTRATION CAN HELP YOU PREVENT LONG-TERM ENERGY DRAINS

It is now scientifically established that practicing Total Concentration on a regular basis can help you

- Get more oxygen into your system
- Control stress
- Relax your muscles completely

The net effect is that your body uses less oxygen. This helps to conserve oxygen for the time when you need more energy. Reduced stress decreases the energy drain on your system and positions you to be more effective in programming yourself to produce more ATP energy molecules.

Your risk of heart disease and the associated conditions of high cholesterol and high blood pressure can be reduced by making adjustments in your diet, lowering your stress level, and exercising daily. Total Concentration helps to magnify the effects of these lifestyle changes. Using the techniques of Total Concentration for as little as ten to fifteen minutes each day can

- Lower your blood pressure
- Reduce your cholesterol level
- Eliminate or reduce the need for blood pressure and cholesterol medication, thus avoiding the extreme tiredness that is often a side effect of some antihypertensive medications
- Improve memory
- Increase creativity

SIX SIMPLE TOTAL CONCENTRATION TECHNIQUES

Below are six easy-to-learn techniques. They all have the same result in terms of improved health. The only difference is in the methodology. Try them all for ten to fifteen minutes each, then pick the one or two methods that you like best:

FOCUS TECHNIQUE #1: THE FIXED IMAGE

With your eyes open, concentrate your attention on a physical object. Mary J. chose to focus on a candle flame. You can just as easily look at a doorknob, a favorite picture, or your hand. Some people like to focus on a religious painting or statue.

FOCUS TECHNIQUE #2: INTERNAL PICTURES

With your eyes closed, concentrate on a mental picture of a physical object. If you will recall, Mary's ritual combined this technique with the fixed image technique; first she stared at the actual candle with her eyes open, then at the "image" of the candle in her mind. In this technique you create a mental image of a single physical object and stare at it with your eyes closed. It doesn't matter what physical object you chose. However, it is important that you don't pick an object or picture that will upset you. Simple objects work best. Some of our clients like to focus on an image of a rose or piece of fruit. Remember that your eyes stay closed. You are looking at an image that your mind creates for you.

FOCUS TECHNIQUE #3: BODY FOCUSING

With your eyes closed, concentrate your attention on a specific part of your body: your heart, nose, big toe, elbow, knee, whatever. There is one exception. If you choose your genitals, you may run the risk of being distracted by other thoughts. Focusing your attention on a specific part of your body is an effective healing technique. It's a way for you to communicate at the subatomic level with the injured or diseased part. This was one of the techniques David used in healing his hernia. He concentrated on "feeling" healing energy vibrations in that area.

FOCUS TECHNIQUE #4: THE NUMBERS GAME

With your eyes closed, concentrate your attention on your breath. Take two or three deep breaths. With the next breath say "one" and hold a picture of the number 1 in your mind's eye as you exhale. Continue breathing deeply and count up to four breaths. Then start over with a count of "one." You may prefer to count up to eight breaths before starting the next sequence. The idea is to stay totally focused during the entire counting process. It's a wonderful technique to train the mind to focus and at the same time relax the body.

FOCUS TECHNIQUE #5: DON'T WAKE THE NEIGHBORS

With your eyes closed, repeat a word or sound over and over again out loud. Some people call this chanting. In this style of total concentration, you try as hard as you can to stay focused on the sound. Depending on how loud you chant and the time of day that you perform, you could get some complaints from neighbors!

FOCUS TECHNIQUE #6: THE SOUND OF SILENCE

With your eyes closed, *silently* repeat a word or sound over and over again. Make no effort to control your thoughts. If your thoughts wander, let them. Then, with no effort, go back to silently repeating the sound. It doesn't matter what word or sound you choose to repeat, although it's wise not to choose an emotionally charged word. Practitioners of transcendental meditation (TM) say you must have a special word, a mantra, given to you by a spiritual leader, for this technique to be effective. If that's their belief, then it is probably true for them since each of us creates his or her own reality. Research, however, shows that a self-chosen word works equally well and offers the same benefits of increased relaxation, decreased stress, improved ability to concentrate, and lowered blood pressure and cholesterol.

SOME TIPS ON TOTAL CONCENTRATION EXERCISES

Almost anyone can do these simple but healthful exercises. If you are taking medication for metabolic or endocrine disorders, for psychiatric reasons, or for the control of pain, you should be monitored by a physician. Medical and psychological research on Total Concentration techniques suggests that people who take medication for the above reasons often have to have their medication reduced and/or eliminated as a result of the process. Assuming that you are not in those categories, you can start these exercises right now. You will get results immediately! However, you should be aware of two other points:

● *Maintain a passive but alert attitude.* Observe your thoughts but don't react to them. You may find all kinds of thoughts coming in and out of your mind. Let your thoughts pass through your mind like fluffy white clouds. Don't resist them. Allow yourself to form a mental picture of them going away. As soon as they are gone, go back to your focusing exercise. Don't *force* your thoughts away; if you do, you will become tense and defeat your purpose.

● *Expect to experience new feelings.* Don't be surprised if you experience strange feelings of warmth, see colors, or sense electricity running up and down your spine. These are perfectly normal feelings. Your unconscious will use this time of rest to get rid of your pent-up emotions and sensations. You may even become sexually aroused. All of these experiences are okay. On the other hand, don't be disappointed if you don't have any of these sensations.

Some people report extrasensory experiences. You can decide what these mean to you if you have them. Remember, your energy consciousness is linked to an infinite network of vibrating strings of energy that make up the universe. Since you will be communicating through this system at the subatomic level, incoming messages are not impossible! David has been doing various forms of meditation and imagery for years. He occasionally has ESP experiences, but he does not seek them, nor are they under his control.

An Extrasensory Experience: David's Story

About two years after my father died suddenly of a heart attack, I moved to Montreal. It was there that I had my first ESP experience. My dad's best friend, who was like a favorite uncle to me, moved to Wisconsin about the same time I moved to Canada. He had been dying of cancer for several years and wanted to return to the place of his birth. His doctors expected him to live at least one or two more years.

One night I went into a deep alpha state and felt the sensation of leaving my body. (Out-of-body experiences are not unusual for many people). I was doing some imagery work, just letting the "pictures" flow across my "imagination screen" when the face of my dad's friend came onto the screen. I silently asked him how he was getting along. He said he was feeling better than he had in years, and added that he had just talked to my father. He said, "Dave, you don't have to worry. Your dad is doing just fine." Then the image faded.

When I came back to a normal state I felt incredibly relaxed and content. Two days later I discovered that on the same night I had this experience my father's best friend had died.

QUICK ENERGY CHARGE #9

A Total Concentration Healing Meditation
Steps 1–5: See the instructions preceding Quick Energy Charge #1 in chapter 4.

Step 6: Energy focusing

Breathing slowly and deeply, see the oxygen entering every cell in your body. See your tiredness and tension melting into the grass, leaving you relaxed and alert. With each breath, breathe in increased energy and breathe out tiredness and stress. See the energy come into your body as pure white light.

Now that your deepest self is tuned in and harmonizing in this relaxed but alert state, allow yourself to be open to the infinite healing energy that is contained in the universe. Begin repeating to yourself as you inhale, "I am" and, as you exhale, "healed."

Continue this process for at least ten minutes. You don't have to time yourself; just estimate the time. If you need to look at a clock, take a peek and continue repeating "I am" as you inhale and "healed" as you exhale.

Step 7: Reentry. See the instructions preceding Quick Energy Charge #1 in chapter 4.

Chapter 17

The Power of Now

Would you like to learn a simple technique that will
- Strengthen your immune system?
- Sharpen your competitive edge?
- Improve your performance?
- Sharpen your perception?
- Improve your communication skills?

Amazing as it sounds, you can gain these benefits by practicing an uncomplicated but extraordinarily powerful technique that focuses total concentration on being in the present. It was demonstrated in a recent popular motion picture, *The Karate Kid*. Daniel, a high school student newly arrived in Los Angeles, is bullied by unethical karate students. Daniel turns for help to Mr. Miyagi, the handyman in his apartment building. Miyagi, it turns out, is an expert in Okinawan karate, a type of martial art that has been handed down in his family for many generations.

The first thing Miyagi does is teach Daniel to wax cars, sand floors, and stain his fence. At first it appears that Miyagi is taking advantage of Daniel, doing a Tom Sawyer number on him. In fact, he is teaching Daniel the real secret of martial arts and one of the most valuable lessons of his—or anyone's—life: *the power of the present moment*. In less than two months of practicing the techniques of total task concentration and body awareness, Daniel learns enough karate skills to win the local championship on his first try.

A LITTLE EFFORT YIELDS BIG DIVIDENDS

Learning to concentrate totally on a single task to the exclusion of all other thoughts and outside stimuli may seem an odd way to strengthen your immune system. You may also wonder how such a technique will also sharpen your perception or communication skills. The fact is, however, that the power of total task concentration—sometimes called *mindfulness* or *the power of now*—is amazing. Let's look at how you can use this power to win some or all of its scientifically established benefits.

YOUR IMMUNE SYSTEM IS STRENGTHENED

When you perform a task, any task, how do you go about it? Do you give it your total concentration? Or are your thoughts everywhere but on the task at hand? These extraneous thoughts often can have stressful overtones. We may be worrying about what happened yesterday or what *might* happen tomorrow. We may be thinking about what people will think about us when and if we finish the task.

Actually, most of us seldom truly live in the present. Most of us live largely in the past and in the future. That's sad, because the past cannot be changed and the future doesn't exist. Yet we spend enormous amounts of mental and emotional energy grappling with these ghosts of the past and phantasms of the future.

The only real time is now, the present moment. Practicing being in the present, focusing on each aspect of what you are doing *now*, helps you relax in a profound and healthful way. It is a form of meditation. Countless experiments prove that relaxation strengthens the immune system while stress tends to weaken it. When you approach a task in a stressful way, your sympathetic nervous system reacts immediately. It mobilizes your muscles and organs into the fight-or-flight stress response: Blood pressure goes up, respiration increases, your heart beats faster, and your muscles tense. Chronic repetition of this syndrome leads to exhaustion and, eventually, to the overload and burnout of your immune system.

In contrast, approaching each task in a more focused way helps your body relax while you are performing. When you are relaxed, blood pressure is lowered, your heart beats more slowly, your muscles are untensed, and your breathing is deeper and slower. Consequently, your immune system is energized by the tasks that you do rather than drained and depleted by them.

YOU CAN SHARPEN YOUR COMPETITIVE EDGE

Any top-flight athlete will tell you that the secret of a good golf shot or tennis stroke is "all in the mind." Besides having a genuine belief in your own ability to win, you must be able to concentrate totally. Coaches have discovered that the practice of total concentration techniques can make the difference between a consistent winner and a frequent loser! So, next time you compete, remember to focus on each element and every detail of the game. We're talking about something beyond just keeping your eye on the ball. We're talking about being totally "present" and aware for every moment of the game.

YOU CAN IMPROVE YOUR PERFORMANCE

When you are totally focused on the task at hand, your power to effect change or perform a skill is beyond what most people consider normal. Nowhere is this power more evident than when a young 120-pound mother physically lifts the wheel of a two-ton automobile off the leg of her baby. You can believe that at that moment the woman was totally focused on the task at hand to the exclusion of all other thoughts! Such "superhuman" feats are more common than you may think. They are extreme examples of the power of being focused on the present task, but they do underscore what is possible for you. The more you practice being totally focused on your task, the more competent you become at performing that task.

YOU CAN SHARPEN YOUR PERCEPTUAL ABILITIES

In studies of men and women who took a three-month course in "mindfulness" training, Harvard psychologist Daniel Brown discovered that perceptual ability can be tremendously heightened. Using a tachistoscope to measure a person's ability to perceive subtle differences in flashes of light, his study showed that with training in mindfulness techniques, subjects could detect flashes of light only one-thousandth of a second apart. For most people these two separate flashes would appear only as a blur of light. But those trained in mindfulness could actually see the gap between the first and second flash!

YOU CAN IMPROVE YOUR COMMUNICATION SKILLS

Donna had at least one phone call a week from her former husband, Peter, to complain about the children's behavior when they were with him. Since the couple had joint custody, it was an especially difficult conversation for Donna. Inevitably, the stress of the calls triggered her fight-or-flight response; her blood pressure rose and her "cramp in the back of the neck" syndrome returned.

After several months of mindfulness training, Donna improved her ability to be totally aware of her physical reactions while concentrating on the task at hand. Thus, when Peter telephoned Donna was able calmly to observe her reactions *as they happened* and to cancel them out mentally so that she could truly concentrate on Peter's words. By focusing totally on what Peter was saying, Donna could now hear Peter's words less as an accusation of her parenting and more as his real concern for the children. Eventually she was able to be more supportive of those concerns and suggest positive ways to deal with them. Donna's new ability to listen intently gradually resulted in a less strained relationship with Peter, and his phone calls became fewer and more pleasant.

TWO WAYS TO GET THE SAME RESULTS

There are two different approaches to mindfulness. Both yield impressive results. You can use them separately or together:

METHOD #1: TOTAL BODY AWARENESS AND OXYGEN PRODUCTION

Jim lies down on the floor of his office twice a day for ten minutes. He concentrates for a minute on his breathing. Then he begins opening himself up to every sensation in his body. He notices the little itch here, the tiny muscle spasm there. He observes these sensations as if he were a fly on the wall. He allows them to enter his consciousness, does not try to block them out. He becomes a detached observer, noticing but not being emotionally attached to his pain, his thoughts, the sounds and sensations of his other bodily functions, or outside noises. He gradually expands his awareness so that he focuses on everything at once.

Although the benefits of practicing this type of mindfulness technique are much the same as the benefits that come from meditation and imagery, the methodology is different. Meditation focuses on a specific object or thought. Imagery concentrates on specific movies of the mind to the exclusion of other thoughts. When you use mindfulness, you open yourself to being totally alert, to focusing on everything at once.

As you will see later on, you can use this technique to stimulate your body to produce more oxygen while you are exercising. The process is similar to visualization. The difference lies in the fact that it is done while you are actually performing a physical task rather than sitting still.

METHOD #2: TOTAL TASK AWARENESS AND OXYGEN CONSERVATION

In a tiny Japanese restaurant in Boston, a porcelain doll–like woman conducts a Japanese tea ceremony. Each movement is a study in the grace, beauty, and power of total task concentration, an effortless flowing of perfection. This young woman practices an age-old Japanese form of mindfulness: total concentration on the skillful performance of even the smallest task. Saint Teresa of Lisieux practiced this same technique as a path to spiritual health and enlightenment. Her credo was that each day of your life you should give your total attention to each task you have to do, each in its turn, no matter how ordinary the chore. St. Teresa believed that whatever you do should be done with the knowledge that it is in harmony with the universe.

When you are able to be this totally aware, two wonderful things happen: First, your body relaxes, thus using less oxygen to perform the task. Since this helps to build your reserves of ATP energy molecules, you will be less tired after you have finished the job. Second, you become extremely adept at whatever you are doing quite quickly.

SAMPLE MINDFULNESS EXERCISES

The first sample exercise will show you how to experience full awareness of your surroundings. The second demonstrates how to focus on a simple task to the complete exclusion of all other thoughts. From these two examples you can develop your own mindfulness exercises.

QUICK ENERGY CHARGE #10

Generating Oxygen

Step 1: Getting comfortable

Choose a spot where you can sit alone in a comfortable chair. Say to yourself, "When I become one with the moment and with nature, I rejuvenate all the cells of my body in this peaceful place."

Step 2: Mind set

Next, take a minute or so to become relaxed. As you inhale, say "So . . ." As you exhale, say "Hum . . ." Repeat these sounds— inhale "Soooooooo," exhale "Hummmmm"—for about five minutes. When you are feeling focused and relaxed, you are ready to open to full awareness of your oneness with the universal energy.

Step 3: Sensing the energy around you

Once you are focused and relaxed, breathe normally. Allow yourself to get in touch with everything in your surroundings. Try to visualize everything in this setting vibrating at the subatomic level. Open all of your senses to the experiences of the moment. Let everything in: the noise of the children playing next door; the passing bus or trolley; if you are outside, the sensation of the cool breeze on your face or the warmth of the sun. Open your eyes and look at the sky. Let the light crossing your optic nerves be the only reality for you at that moment. Then listen to the sounds in your body: the silent vibrations of your digestive tract; the gentle pulsing of blood flowing through your brain. Continue to fill yourself with all the thoughts, feelings, sensations, and experiences of being in your particular surroundings at this very moment.

Do not *judge* your thoughts or your physical sensations. Keep a passive attitude about any and all thoughts that enter your mind. Let them pass through your mind gently. Continue to pay total attention to everything, all at once. Like a fly on the wall, remain detached. Observe but don't react to any emotional responses or to any sensations. Just notice them and let them be.

It is most important that you carry with you throughout this total awareness experience the belief that *this particular moment is the most important moment of your life.* Also carry the belief that *being here in this moment puts you in complete harmony with the energy vibrations of the universe.*

Step 4: Energy programming

Now that your body and mind are totally aware, you should feel relaxed. Use you mind's flashlight to illuminate each and every cell in your body. Say to yourself, "Because I am relaxed, my blood is full of oxygen. Therefore, my cells are creating more and more high-energy molecules (ATP) in a never-ending stream. I become stronger and healthier every time I focus on what I am doing." Sense the subtle difference in your energy level.

QUICK ENERGY CHARGE #11

A High-Energy Shower

Step 1: Mind set

As you step into the shower, say to yourself, "When I shower, I cleanse my body and mind of all impurities." Next, take a minute or so to relax. As you inhale, say "So . . ." As you exhale, say "Hum . . ." Repeat this phrase—inhale "Soooooooo," exhale "Hummmmm"—over and over. When you are feeling focused and relaxed, you are ready to open yourself to the task of showering.

Step 2: Sensing the energy around you

Once you are focused and relaxed, begin focusing your energy consciousness on the task of showering. Feel the warmth of the water on your back. Listen intently to the sound of the water as it hits your skin. Notice the physcial sensations as each drop runs down your back and legs. Continue to open yourself up to all the sensations in your environment. Notice the hum of the exhaust fan, the sound of passing automobiles and other outside noises. Hold all these sensations in your consciousness. Next, pick up the soap. Feel its slipperiness. Smell its fragrance. Begin scrubbing your body with the bar of soap. Notice the various muscles in your body as you scrub. Be alert to every move you make to cleanse your body. Remember, your purpose is to be totally focused on the task, to experience the moment at its fullest. When conflicting thoughts enter your mind, notice them. Say, "Isn't that interesting that I thought of that," and let the thought go by.

Do not judge your thoughts or your physical sensations. Keep a passive attitude about any interfering thoughts that are not task-focused. Let them pass through your mind gently. Then go back to paying total attention to every move you make to complete the task of washing your body in the shower. Feel at this moment that this task is the most important thing in your life.

Step 3: Energy programming
When you finish showering, use your mind's flashlight to illuminate each and every cell in your body. Say to yourself, "Because I am relaxed, my blood is full of oxygen. Therefore, my cells are creating more and more high-energy molecules (ATP) in a never-ending stream. I get stronger and healthier every time I focus on what I am doing." Sense the subtle difference in your energy level. Say to yourself, "I feel wonderful every time I shower like this!"

Part IV

ENERGY-BUILDING EXERCISES

Chapter 18

Create Energy: Burn Oxygen

You'd have to be an ostrich with your head in the sand not to know that exercise is good for you. "I know, I know," we can hear you saying. "It's supposed to be good for me, but I don't like it. It doesn't feel good, and I don't want to do it." That may be your current reality, but was it always like that? Surely you remember those early years when you took such joy in running, jumping, climbing, swinging, digging, skating, swimming, diving, playing ball. What happened to you? What happened to your body? And more important, what happened to your mind that it has changed an experience that is completely joyous into something to be avoided at all costs?

Make no mistake about it. Your mind controls your body. Why then did you choose to see yourself as an adult whose arduous responsibilities leave no time for your body to experience the joy of movement. The effect of this choice was to make you a conspirator in the gradual deterioration of your body. And, based on the use-it-or-lose-it school of thought, please believe that your body *is* deteriorating. In addition, you are not getting the increased ATP production that is an integral part and result of cardiovascular exercise. The end result: a low energy level.

EXCUSES FOR NOT EXERCISING

People offer two common excuses for not exercising. One is "I don't like it." The other is "I don't have the time." If the latter is your excuse, take a closer look at how valid it is by answering the following two questions.

TIME MANAGEMENT QUIZ

1. If we asked you to spend an extra half hour at work, and in return guaranteed you greater productivity, better problem-solving skills, more energy, and positive relationships with your coworkers, would you do it?
2. If we asked you to spend an extra half hour at home, and in return guaranteed you would have more patience with the kids, more energy, and therefore more time to spend with them, would you do it?

Without exception, everyone in our seminars has said yes to one if not both of these questions.

Did you say yes to either of them? If so, why is it that you have a half hour to give to your company or a half hour to give to your children but you don't have a half hour to give to yourself?

The irony is that all the benefits we listed for work or home will accrue, willy-nilly, when you give that half hour of exercise to yourself!

Another way you can look at exercise is as an investment in yourself. No doubt you have spent years preparing for your future. You went to school, you work hard at your job, you manage your money wisely. How about investing a little time to make sure you *have* a future? How about putting some energy now into making sure that your future is a relaxed and vibrant one?

EXERCISE, OXYGEN, AND ENERGY

The fitness revolution in America is not just about looking good, losing weight, or protecting against heart disease. *The fitness revolution is about having more energy available every single day,* more than you ever thought possible. It's about never being tired again. It's about sleeping like a log and then getting up in the morning knowing you'll have all the energy you need to get you through your day feeling good. It's about making your life more productive. You can create this high level of energy for yourself naturally by burning oxygen at a faster rate. As you will recall from our discussion in chapter 4, this is what happens when you exercise cardiovascularly. And when you burn oxygen at this faster rate, your body naturally produces more of the ATP energy-storage molecules. The result: You are building incredible reserves of energy that will be there when you need them—for work, for play, for recreation, for making love.

Matt's Experience

Matt, a publishing executive, is a graduate of our live-in program. During the time he spent with us he told us what happened to his employees when he started an incentive program for them. As part of the program he offered to pay a generous portion of the cost of a health club membership. In addition to the motivational aspects of the free membership, he anticipated that participating employees would get the health benefits he had heard so much about.

Matt's employees did get all of these. But the unanticipated dividend for his company was an immediate and astonishing jump in the productivity of the exercising employees! Not only were they more productive, Matt pointed out, they were also easier to work with. They were calmer, friendlier, and dealt better with pressure. "And in my business," Matt said, "that's essential if you want to succeed."

CARDIOVASCULAR EXERCISE DEFINED

Scientifically defined, an aerobic activity (cardiovascular exercise) is any kind of physical motion that requires you to use a lot of oxygen over a sustained period of time. The ability of your lungs to handle oxygen under this kind of stress is called your *vital capacity*, and it is a powerful predictor of longevity. For practical purposes, our definition of cardiovascular (or aerobic) exercise translates into meeting four conditions.

FOUR KEY CONDITIONS THAT MAKE AN EXERCISE CARDIOVASCULAR

1. *The exercise is steady and nonstop.* This means that you do not stop moving from the time you begin until the time the exercise ends.
2. *You maintain a heart rate that is 70 to 80 percent of your maximum heart rate.* We call this your energy-building heart rate (EBHR). You can determine your own energy-building heart rate using a simple formula explained in the next chapter.

These first two conditions would probably mean that activities like a doubles tennis game would not qualify as cardiovascular exercise. Unless you play at a professional level, you probably move quickly only for brief periods of time; for most of the match you're going to be standing around waiting to make a shot or watching your partner run. This means that your heart rate would drop below 70 to 80 percent of its maximum.

3. *The activity continues for at least fifteen minutes at your energy-building heart rate.* Although twelve minutes is scientifically correct, it represents an average figure. We recommend that you consider fifteen minutes as the minimum time to be at this rate of cardiovascular activity. Fifteen minutes gives you a safety cushion, and insures maximum benefits. This minimum period *does not* include the time you need to get your heart rate up and pumping. This takes about five minutes if you are jogging or riding a stationary bike. Bottom line: You need to invest *twenty minutes* if you are going to jog or use a stationary bike. Swimming and brisk walking require a total investment of thirty minutes. You also need to add a five- to ten-minute cool-down period to allow your heart rate to return to normal.

4. *You exercise a minimum of four days a week.* Four days a week will keep you cardiovascularly fit, but if you want to lose weight and keep it off you must exercise five days a week.

THE PHYSICAL BENEFITS OF CARDIOVASCULAR EXERCISE

● *Your heart muscle becomes thicker and stronger.*

The more you exercise, the more oxygen your heart must pump to your muscles. To meet this increased demand, your heart beats faster during exercise. And like any other muscle that is exercised, it will become stronger. Cardiovascular exercise also helps arteries relax and be more pliable; they may actually increase in diameter, thus reducing their resistance to the flow of blood. The end result is a lessened risk of heart attack. In almost all cases, heart disease can be prevented with exercise, good nutrition, and the use of quick energy charges.

- *Your pulse rate slows.*

As your heart becomes larger and stronger, it beats more slowly because it is able to pump more blood with each stroke. Therefore, your pulse slows down. Generally, the slower your pulse, the more cardiovascularly fit you are. The difference between being physically fit and unfit can mean 30,000 fewer heartbeats a day! In addition to saving wear and tear on your heart, this makes more energy available for the rest of your physical needs.

- *Your blood pressure normalizes.*

More than 80 million Americans suffer from high blood pressure. Antihypertensives are among the most prescribed medications. Their many side effects include an increased cholesterol level, chronic tiredness, and, for some men, impotence. High blood pressure itself can damage the kidneys, the eyes, even the brain. For most people, cardiovascular exercise is a natural way to lower blood pressure and maintain it within a normal range *without* medication.

- *Your cholesterol levels are reduced.*

Exercise raises your level of high-density lipoprotein (HDL), known as "good cholesterol" because it helps keep fat from building up in your arteries, thus preventing heart disease and stroke.

- *You can lose weight permanently.*

We know that your body "defends" its weight when you reduce the number of calories you take in by more than 500 calories a day. This defense mechanism is called the "set point." According to set point theory, dieting alone will not get rid of excess weight. However, regular exercise can lower your set point, increase your metabolism, and help keep weight off permanently.

OTHER PHYSICAL PLUSES

- The aging process is slowed down as the increased oxygen intake postpones cellular degeneration.
- Blood has less tendency to clot.
- Energy increases.
- Digestion improves.
- Bowels function better.
- Appetite is brought into line with your body's needs.
- Sex drive increases.
- Body temperature rises by several degrees while exercising; this helps to kill bacteria.

- Increased sensitivity to insulin is a real benefit to diabetics.
- Running in particular prevents calcium loss in bones. This guards against osteoporosis, which can start around age thirty-five and affects 30 percent of women and 10 percent of men over sixty. Half of all people over seventy have it!

THE PSYCHOLOGICAL BENEFITS OF CARDIOVASCULAR EXERCISE

- *Exercise helps control depression.* Many psychiatrists and psychologists prescribe daily cardiovascular exercise as a natural way to control depression in patients.
- *Exercise helps control stress.* There are several theories as to why this happens. Some experts believe exercise stimulates certain brain hormones, such as beta-endorphins, which produce a sense of well-being and lowered anxiety. Still others say it's due to the brain's increased blood supply.

Regardless of the reason, our experience supports the fact that it works. In our private practice we specialize in helping people with stress-associated problems. Our first recommendation invariably is an appropriate cardiovascular exercise program (assuming the patient has clearance from a physician). We find there is no substitute for the incredible sense of well-being and calmness that comes from exercise. And it has none of the negative side effects of the pill-popping approach to stress control.

- *Exercise improves self-concept.* Have you noticed the difference between people who are fit and those who are not? Generally, the physically fit carry themselves straighter and taller. They are more likely to take on challenges, to exhibit more energy and enthusiasm. These factors, the natural result of regular exercise, help strengthen one's self-concept.
- *Exercise increases mental productivity.* Nobody knows exactly why, but most likely the increase is due to the increase in oxygen-rich blood in the brain. Matt, whose story we recounted earlier, saw this result in his employees. A number of studies show that exercise also improves problem-solving skills and enhances original thinking.

Chapter 19 gives the information you need to begin an exercise program. Chapter 20 describes in detail basic exercise programs that you can individualize to meet your personal needs.

QUICK ENERGY CHARGE #12

Burn Energy, Burn Oxygen

Steps 1–5. See the instructions preceding Quick Energy Charge #1 in chapter 4.

Step 6: Energy programming

Breathing slowly and deeply, see the oxygen entering every cell in your body. See your tiredness and tension melting into the grass, leaving you relaxed and alert. With each breath, breathe in increased energy and breathe out tiredness and stress. See the energy come into your body as pure white light.

Now that your deepest self is tuned in and harmonizing in this relaxed but alert state, ask your deepest self to choose the "elegant solution" for getting more energy by burning oxygen every time you exercise. Say to every cell, every vibrating energy string in your body, "I have chosen to get more energy by burning oxygen. Each time I get involved in physical activity I create more and more high energy molecules (ATP). With each passing day I am more physically fit."

Shine your mind's flashlight on every cell in your body. See your cells manufacturing an endless stream of high-energy molecules (ATP) that nourish and rejuvenate each and every cell. See in your mind's eye your body's glucose combining with the extra oxygen your exercise program generates. Look into the imaginary mirror of your mind and see yourself growing younger, stronger, and more energetic with each passing day. Follow that thought deep into the mirror of your mind and beyond.

Clear your mind of all other thoughts except the picture of the younger, stronger, more energetic You in the mirror. Notice how comfortable you feel with this image of yourself. Let the fundamental energy vibrations that are you sense the permanence of your lifestyle decision, to be always in this high-energy level of being.

Step 7: Reentry. See the instructions preceding Quick Energy Charge #1 in chapter 4.

How to Start Your High-Energy Exercise Program

By now, we hope, you are so enthusiastic you're ready to start exercising immediately and go all out.

Don't—especially if you are over thirty.

Unless you start your exercise program correctly, you may end up with serious medical problems. Please do not begin your cardiovascular exercise program until you have read and followed the instructions in this chapter. Then you may choose from the recommended exercises.

Warning: Before beginning any exercise program it is essential that you consult your physician and have a complete physical examination, including a stress test for your heart.

HOW TO DETERMINE YOUR ENERGY-BUILDING HEART RATE (EBHR)

Pushing your heart too hard and too fast can be dangerous. At the same time, not excercising hard enough means there will be little or no physiological benefit. Your first goal, then, is to establish a safe *and* effective exercise heart rate for yourself. We call this the "energy-building heart rate." It is also called the "training heart rate," but we think "energy-building" is a more positive and accurate description.

If you have a health problem, ask your physician to recommend a safe exercise heart rate for you. If you are in good health, you can establish your own safe EBHR by following the steps below.

1. Subtract your age from 220 if you are a man, and from 226 if you are a woman.

2. Multiply the result by 70 percent if you have not exercised in the past year, and by 80 percent if you are already on a regular exercise program. The resulting figure is your EBHR—the number of times your heart should beat during sixty seconds of exercise to get the most benefit from your workouts. This is the rate at which you can exercise safely and at the same time force your cardiovascular system to become stronger.

3. Since it is hard to take your pulse for full sixty seconds while working out, a short-cut is to determine the rate for ten seconds. Simply divide your energy-building heart rate by 6.

EXAMPLE OF THE FORMULA FOR MEN

Dave is fifty-four years old. His energy-building heart rate is calculated as follows:

Dave's EBHR $= 220 - 54 = 166 \times .80^* = 133$
Dave's 10-second EBHR $= 133 \div 6 = 22$

*Remember to use .70 if you haven't been exercising.

EXAMPLE OF THE FORMULA FOR WOMEN

Joely is forty-one years old. Her energy-building heart rate is calculated as follows:

Joely's EBHR $= 226 - 41 = 185 \times .80^* = 148$
Joely's 10-second EBHR $= 148 \div 6 = 24$

*Remember to use .70 if you haven't been exercising.

Reminder: Do not start an exercise program without your physician's approval and without having had a complete physical examination.

HOW TO TAKE YOUR OWN PULSE

Place your index and middle fingers on the inside of your wrist or on the side of your throat just under your jaw line, or put your hand over your heart. Count the number of beats for ten seconds. Then multiply by 6. If you have trouble finding your pulse, get a friend to help you find it.

It really is important to check your pulse. One man we know thought he was getting a terrific workout until he checked his pulse and found it was considerably lower than it should be. He had spent months exercising at a nonaerobic rate! Of course he gained some benefits—he burned calories and got rid of some fat—but he didn't get the heart-building benefits he could have. There are many pulse monitors on the market today, from watches to digital readout devices. Invest in one if you think it will help you check your pulse rate more accurately.

NINE BASIC STEPS TO A SUCCESSFUL ENERGY-BUILDING EXERCISE PROGRAM

You are now ready to choose and schedule your high-energy program. Remember, you must exercise at least four days a week to maintain cardiovascular fitness, and at least five days a week to establish permanent weight loss. Here are nine practical guidelines on how to do it:

1. PICK YOUR OWN BEST TIME FOR EXERCISE

Personally, we find that we get too involved in our work to stop and exercise before dinner. So we make a point of exercising in the morning. That way we make sure we do it. Although it's true that you have to get up earlier in order to fit in your workout, it's also true that regular cardiovascular exercise increases your energy level. In the long run, the benefits of cardiovascular activity will far outweigh the effort that goes into doing it.

Fitting Kids into an Exercise Schedule

When David's two children were younger, we let them ride their bikes alongside us while we jogged. Now that they are a little older, they often walk or jog with us. It's a good way to get them involved, and it gives them a chance to see that physical abilities do not need to deteriorate with age.

Ted, a graduate of our program, does the same thing with his two sons of nine and five. Before Ted encouraged them to take part in his exercise routine, getting them to go to bed was a real source of conflict. The boys were staying up later and later. As a result, Ted and his wife had little private time. After Ted started taking the boys with him on his morning jog in the park, they were more than ready for bed at a decent time. In addition, the boys like the idea of having a "special time" with their dad. Ted and his wife like having extra time to be alone together.

2. PICK TWO ALTERNATIVES

Some people look for any excuse to cop out of their workout schedule. Usually it's the weather: "Can't bike, it's snowing" . . . "Can't walk, it's raining." One man told us he couldn't do his swim laps because his pool was being drained. We therefore recommend that you pick *two* exercise activities, to give you an option. For example, if you're a power walker and it's icy out, you can still swim in an indoor pool. Having two workout alternatives also cuts down on the risk of boredom.

Note from Dave

One of the basic appeals of exercise for me is that it is so cost effective in terms of personal input versus personal gain. For a minimum investment of time you can harvest the mental and physical benefits we listed earlier. And this can happen in as little as eighty minutes a week, depending on the type of exercise you choose. If you run or use a bicycle exerciser twenty minutes a day, you are using only a bit more than 1 percent of the total time available to you in a week. Even if you add dressing time and a five-minute cool-down, you are still well under 2 percent of your available time per week.

3. TAKE IT SLOW AND EASY

Work up to fitness gradually. As you meet each short-term fitness goal, you will be more motivated to continue. Invariably in our private practice and with our live-in training groups there is always at least one "gung ho" personality who believes that if some exercise is good, then more is better. Within a day or so the "machos" (and they can and do include women!) are out of the game with blisters, sore and cramping muscles, or an injury. The name of the game is slow and easy!

4. WRITE DOWN YOUR PROGRAM GOALS

Psychologists have studied the effects of goal-setting on be-havior for over fifty years. Among the many things they learned is that if you write down your goals you are more likely to achieve them. You are more likely to stick with your Never Be Tired Again exercise program if you write down your exercise goals. Include times, days of the week, and duration. Some people need charts, graphs, targets, etc. to motivate themselves. If you have a computer, try motivating yourself with a software program that prints out graphs and charts of your daily progress.

5. MAKE YOUR NEW HABIT A REGULAR ONE

Do your exercises every day at the same time. This helps you to become psychologically and physiologically accustomed to the routine. Never skip more than one day unless you are genuinely ill. It's much too easy, particularly in the beginning, to go back to your old sedentary ways.

Positive Addiction Pays Off

One of our former graduates has a treadmill in his master bed-room suite. He has a reading stand and a remote control VCR/TV setup. He uses one or both of them while he exercises on the treadmill for forty-five minutes every morning before breakfast. Sometimes he reads for pleasure, sometimes for business; or he watches TV news or a videocassette movie. He claims he never is bored. More important, in the first five months on our program he lost thirty-five pounds, even though he claims he has never eaten so much in his life!

6. CHOOSE MEASURABLE CARDIOVASCULAR EXERCISES

The psychological reason for making your primary workout activity a measurable one is that you must be able to see progress if you expect to stay motivated. Your job is to get your body fit enough so that it will protest when you *don't* exercise! There are other ways to get cardiovascularly fit besides the ones we recom-mend in the next chapter, but they are harder to quantify. For example, it's easy to quantify walking by time and distance; it's not easy to quantify activities such as tennis or racquetball. Use them as your secondary or alternate forms of exercise.

7. DON'T GET COMPETITIVE

We do not recommend competitive sports as a primary form of exercise. One of the benefits of our Never Be Tired Again exercise program is that the activities we suggest have been shown to reduce stress. It seems counterproductive to add another competitive situation to your already stressful life.

8. HAVE FUN DOING IT!

Finding ways to have fun while keeping yourself cardiovascularly fit is limited only by your own imagination and attitude. Jog with friends and make it a social occasion. Watch movies while you are on the treadmill. Read while on the stationary bicycle. Go cross-country skiing or take long mountain hikes with your family. Work out with friends at the club. If you don't find a way to make exercise fun, you will have difficulty sticking with any workout program.

9. REWARD YOURSELF

Set up lots of short-term goals and rewards. Don't slip back into old habit patterns and choose a reward that is in conflict with your goal. For example, don't reward yourself with a hot fudge sundae after meeting your first exercise goal. Treat yourself to a great-looking exercise outfit or a membership in a club, or sign up for tennis lessons (or some other activity you've always wanted to learn). You deserve it!

QUICK ENERGY CHARGE #13

Programming Goals
Steps 1–5. See the instructions preceding Quick Energy Charge #1 in chapter 4.

Step 6: Energy programming
Breathing slowly and deeply, see the oxygen entering every cell in

your body. See your tiredness and tension melting into the grass, leaving you relaxed and alert. With each breath, breathe in increased energy and breathe out tiredness and stress. See the energy come into your body as pure white light.

Now that your deepest self is tuned in and harmonizing in this relaxed but alert state, ask your Energy Consciousness to help you plan your exercise program. Keeping your eyes closed, imagine that you are looking at a large white movie screen. See yourself walking up and onto the stage in front of the screen. Write on it in big black letters this heading: THE WAY I AM GOING TO HANDLE MY EXERCISE PROGRAM. Then begin printing your list of exercise goals in large, black print on this screen. Start with the number 1. Print: 1. GET A PHYSICAL EXAMINATION ON *(date)*. Next, see yourself printing your second goal: 2. *(you fill in the goal)*.

When you have finished printing your initial list of exercise goals on your imaginary screen, take time to go over in your mind each goal in detail. Make a mental note of any problems you think may be a barrier to accomplishing these goals. Each time a "barrier thought" enters your mind, let it pass across the white screen but don't write it down. Instead write down a solution on the large white screen that clears away each and every barrier. Continue this process until it feels complete.

Step 7: Reentry. See the instructions preceding Quick Energy Charge # 1 in chapter 4.

Chapter 20

Effective Exercises for Cardiovascular Fitness

There are a variety of ways to achieve and/or maintain cardiovascular fitness. In this chapter we will discuss the advantages and drawbacks of the four basic Never Be Tired Again lifestyle exercise programs: walking, swimming, biking, and running/jogging. We'll provide you with a start-up plan for each, and show you how to tailor that plan to accommodate your personal fitness level.

Whichever high-energy exercise program you choose, be sure it meets as many of the following standards as possible:
- The activity should get your heartbeat up to 70 to 80 percent of its capacity.
- You should be able to fit the activity into your daily schedule without having to do a major juggling act.
- You should not need a lot of equipment or any special skill in order to do the exercise.
- You should be able to do the exercise alone or with other people.
- The activity should be measurable. That is, you must be able to check your progress against scientifically established aerobic fitness standards. You should also be able to tell how much progress you are making by noting the improvement in your own time-versus-distance records.

The closer your program matches these criteria, the easier it will be for you to get started, to see immediate results, and to stick with the program.

You shouldn't think of your exercise program as an unpleasant or even hateful chore. If you haven't been exercising recently, your body is going to rebel. There is a principle in physics called the Law of Entropy, which says that any system left to itself tends to decay over time. When you don't regularly use your muscle system it decays over time.

The following exercise programs were chosen on the basis of the criteria listed above. Not all of them meet all five criteria, but their advantages outweigh their disadvantages. Swimming, for example, requires equipment (a pool) but has the advantage of exercising your whole body with minimum risk of injury. Walking and running/jogging do meet all the criteria, but running has some disadvantages, the most serious being the risk of injury. Fast walking is probably the best all-around choice for most people, but you need to do it longer than most of the other activities to obtain the same physical benefits. As noted earlier, we suggest you choose a primary activity and an alternate activity.

TIMING IS EVERYTHING

Our friend Peter, a senior partner in a major accounting firm and a heck of a nice fellow, also can be stubborn. Peter has adult-onset diabetes and high blood pressure. He should exercise to control his ailments but insisted that his frantically busy schedule didn't leave time for it. Because he often had to visit his firm's district offices, there were many days when Peter had to get up even earlier than usual. As far as he was concerned, this eliminated morning exercise, and he was frantically busy all day and into the evening.

One day Peter told us that he always watched the 10 P.M. news. Eureka! Peter now has an exercise bike in front of his television set. He can exercise for thirty minutes four or five times a week without feeling "pressured" by another addition to his day's schedule. By combining regular exercise with the nutrition program outlined later in this book, Peter brought his blood pressure and blood sugar levels down to normal for the first time in years, and he's lost weight.

YOUR PERSONAL HIGH-ENERGY WALKING PROGRAM

The basic drawback to walking is that it requires more time to get cardiovascular benefits than many other exercises. If time is not an issue for you, walking may well be the most enjoyable form of cardiovascular exercise. In addition, it is usually the perfect program for many people with health problems.

ADVANTAGES OF A HIGH-ENERGY WALKING PROGRAM

- Almost everyone can walk, no matter how old you are or what shape you're in.
- You don't need any particular equipment, just a good pair of walking shoes.
- There is an extremely low risk of injury.
- You can walk by yourself, with another person, and even in walking clubs.

One of the newest fitness techniques to win popularity is fast walking, or race walking. Advocates claim it has distinct advantages over ordinary walking or running. The primary advantage is that the hip-swaying stride of race walking causes more pelvic rotation, which in turn helps strengthen the lower abdominal muscles that keep the pelvis level, the back strong, and the tummy flat. Whether you decide on race walking or plain, old-fashioned walking, the charts below offer guidelines.

AEROBIC FITNESS RATING FOR WALKING

Pace of Activity	Calories Burned		Aerobic Fitness Rating
	20 mins.	30 mins.	
Walking 1 mile in 30 min.	50	75	None
Walking 1 mile in 20 min.	80	120	Low. This is for people who can't exercise vigorously.
Walking 1 mile in 17 min.	100	150	Medium
Fast walking 1 mile in 15 min.	120–140	180–210	High
Fast walking 1 mile in 12 min.	160	240	High

YOUR PERSONAL HIGH-ENERGY WALKING START-UP PLAN

Below are two start-up plans for people who are in good health. Plan I is for men and women under thirty-five, and for those who have been exercising already and want a more vigorous workout. Plan II is for those over thirty-five. Remember, don't begin either program—even if you are healthy—without the approval of your physician. If your physician feels these plans are too strenuous for you, ask for a modified plan. It is perfectly all right to start out slowly and build up to physical fitness. The important thing is that you start moving no matter what the pace!

PLAN I:
PERSONAL START-UP PLAN FOR WALKING
(Healthy, Under 35)

WEEKLY GOALS

Step	What to Do	Times per Wk.*	Miles	Mins. per Mile	Flexibility** (Mins.)	Total Hrs.:Mins. per Wk.
1	Walk	5 (5)	1.0	17	20	3:05
2	Walk	3 (5)	2.0	17	20	2:42
3	Walk	4 (5)	2.0	16	20	3:28
4	Fast Walk	5	2.0	15	20	4:10
5	Fast Walk	5	2.5	15	20	4:48
6	Fast Walk	5	2.5	14.5	20	4:41
7	Fast Walk	5	2.5	14	20	4:35
8	Fast Walk	5	3.0	15	20	5:25
9	Fast Walk	5	3.0	14.8	20	5:22
10	Fast Walk	5	3.0	14.5	20	5:18
11	Fast Walk	4 (5)	3.0	14	20	4:08
12	Fast Walk	5	3.0	14	20	5:10

*If you want to do the seven-day program outlined in chapter 10, make sure you have your doctor's okay first. We discovered in our live-in program that weight loss was accelerated by additional daily workout sessions during the start-up period. When you are at your cardiovascular fitness level, as shown in the plan for the tenth week, you must continue to exercise a minimum of thirty minutes per day, five days per week, to permanently impact your set point.

**If you want to reduce muscle soreness and prevent injury, we recommend the flexibility program in the following chapter.

Once you have selected the appropriate plan (over thirty-five or under thirty-five), your next decision should be how often you will exercise each week. Under the "Times per Week" column on the Personal Start-Up Plan for Walking, the first number is what we recommend if you are primarily concerned with aerobic fitness. The number in parentheses is the recommended number of times to exercise if you also want to lose weight. To do that you need to work out more frequently in order to affect your set point. In addition, both the over-thirty-five and under-thirty-five plans include the recommended number of minutes of flexibility training that should be part of your balanced workout program. So the indicated total hours or minutes per week include the amount of

PLAN II:
PERSONAL START-UP PLAN FOR WALKING
(Healthy, Over 35)
WEEKLY GOALS

Step	What to Do	Times per Wk.*	Miles	Mins. per Mile	Flexibility** (Mins.)	Total Hrs.:Mins. per Wk.
1	Walk	5 (14)	1.0	18	20	3:10
2	Walk	3 (5)	2.0	18	20	2:48
3	Walk	3 (5)	2.0	17	20	2:42
4	Walk	4 (5)	2.0	16	20	3:28
5	Walk	5	2.0	15	20	4:10
6	Walk	4 (5)	2.5	15.6	20	3:56
7	Walk	5	2.5	15.2	20	4:50
8	Fast Walk	5	2.5	15	20	4:48
9	Fast Walk	5	3.0	15.5	20	5:33
10	Fast Walk	5	3.0	15	20	5:25
11	Fast Walk	4 (5)	3.0	14.5	20	4:14
12	Fast Walk	5	3.0	14.5	20	5:18

*If you want to do the seven-day program outlined in chapter 10, make sure you have your doctor's okay first. We discovered in our live-in program that weight loss was accelerated by additional daily workout sessions during the start-up period. When you are at your cardiovascular fitness level, as shown in the plan for the tenth week, you must continue to exercise a minimum of thirty minutes per day, five days per week, to permanently impact your set point.

**If you want to reduce muscle soreness and prevent injury, we recommend the flexibility program in the next chapter.

exercise time required for cardiovascular fitness *plus* twenty minutes a day, five days a week, for flexibility.

You can upgrade to running at any time. For example, if you are over thirty-five and have completed and maintained step 12 in the over-thirty-five start-up plan, you can easily go to a fourteen-minute mile without too much effort if your body tells you that it's ready. *A word of caution:* If you have chosen walking as your primary aerobic activity because of a physical problem or on the advice of your physician, be careful about upgrading to running/jogging. Don't do it without your doctor's approval. Swimming or biking may be better alternatives or complementary activities.

The Treadmill as a Walking Option
Note from Joely

I really like walking on a treadmill. The new treadmills have all kinds of gadgets that allow you to speed them up or slow them down at the touch of a button, or to increase the incline so you're walking uphill. You can thus get a terrific workout no matter what your level of fitness.

This really worked out well for one particular couple. Leonard was in better physical condition than his wife, Helen. He was extremely solicitous of her, and when we walked outdoors he always stayed close to her, matching his pace to hers to make sure she was all right. Because Helen's pace was so much slower than Leonard's, he did not get any cardiovascular conditioning from the exercise. Treadmills solved the problem. The couple could work out alongside each other, yet each could go at his or her own pace. At the beginning of the program, Helen literally could not walk for five minutes. At the end of the program she was walking for thirty minutes.

A treadmill can be a real boon in bad weather. I know from experience that it takes incredible motivation to get up and out when it's extremely cold or hot or rainy. I have to confess that David is the one with the motivation in these instances. I go along only because I'd feel too guilty waving goodbye from my nice warm (or dry or cool) house. Of course, I have to admit I always feel better (and certainly more virtuous) when I finish exercising, no matter what the weather is like.

If time is important to you or if you find exercise unutterably boring, consider a treadmill. If you can walk and chew gum at the same time, you're in business. The real reason I like the treadmill so much is that I have learned to read while walking. This gives me a solid half hour of uninterrupted reading pleasure. While reading a really good book, at times I've walked for forty-five to fifty minutes without realizing it. I guess if you're a classic Type A, you could even read for business.

One of our graduates rents movies for his VCR and watches while treadmilling. He gets through a movie every two days. Television is another possible diversion. Most of the time-use benefits that you can obtain from treadmills are also obtainable when using exercise bikes.

A HIGH-ENERGY SWIMMING PROGRAM

Swimming is probably the best all-around cardiovascular fitness exercise because it exercises the upper and lower body at the same time. The force of gravity is held in check in the water, thus virtually eliminating the risk of injury. Swimming doesn't put any wear and tear on joints and tendons. On top of all these benefits, swimming is a "no sweat" activity, and most people associate it psychologically with "summer fun." There is also a calorie burn-off factor. Did you know that your body cools twenty-five times faster in water than in air? So even though you're working hard, it doesn't really feel like it!

ADVANTAGES OF A HIGH-ENERGY SWIMMING PROGRAM

- You exercise all major muscles as well as your upper and lower body.
- There is less risk of injury than in any other aerobic activity.
- There is less strain on joints and bones.
- Poolside offers a lot of social opportunities.
- It can be competitive or not—your choice.
- You can combine it with other activities—snorkeling, scuba diving, beach picnics, etc.

In addition, a high-energy swimming program carries a high aerobic fitness rating because it makes your heart stronger, and it increases your vital capacity by making your lungs more efficient. Swimming strictly for pleasure as opposed to swimming for exercise does not provide the same benefits.

AEROBIC FITNESS RATING FOR SWIMMING

Pace of Activity	Calories Burned		Aerobic Fitness Rating
	20 mins.	30 mins.	
Swimming (pleasure)	120	180	Medium
Swimming 1 lap* in 1 min. 36 sec.	160	240	High
Swimming 1 lap in 1 min. 15 sec.	220	330	High
Swimming 1 lap in 1 min.	250	375	High

*One lap is one round trip in an Olympic-size pool, or a total of fifty yards.

Who Is That Masked Woman?
Note from Joely

I was not an especially good swimmer when I started. I hated putting my face into the water, probably because I never learned to breathe properly while swimming. Consequently, I went through several months of straining to keep my head out of the water. Naturally, I didn't make much progress. Then we started taking scuba lessons. First we had to practice using the scuba mask and snorkel in the pool. What a difference! I could breathe without having to twist my head back and forth. Now I won't swim without my mask and snorkel. A good diving shop is the best place to go to get properly fitted. A good mask can cost from $35 to $70, but for me it was well worth it. Our kids enjoy the masks, which are now standard equipment when we go to the beach.

Even Our Hairdresser Doesn't Know for Sure
Note from Dave

When we first started living the Never Be Tired Again lifestyle, we used swimming as our primary workout. In the beginning I found that my hair was not only bleaching out but was getting dry. The chlorine in a public pool can do a number on your skin and hair. I made an effort to check out all the "natural" hair conditioners in the health food store. I finally found one that works beautifully. It is made from aloe, jojoba, and a natural coconut fatty acid base. Within a week, my hairstylist couldn't believe the change. From then on, there was no problem even if I swam every day. If you swim regularly, make an investment in good skin creams and hair conditioners.

YOUR PERSONAL HIGH-ENERGY SWIMMING START-UP PLAN

Below are two start-up plans for people in good health. Plan I is for men and women under thirty-five, and for those who have been exercising already and want a more vigorous workout. Plan II is for those over thirty-five. Remember, don't begin either of these programs—even if you are healthy—without the approval of your physician. If your physician feels these plans are too strenuous for you, ask for a modified plan. It's perfectly all right to start out slowly and build up to physical fitness. The important thing is that you start moving, no matter what your pace!

PLAN I:
PERSONAL START-UP PLAN FOR SWIMMING
(Healthy, Under 35)
WEEKLY GOALS

Step	What to Do	Times per Wk.*	No. of Laps	Time per Lap	Flexibility** (mins.)	Total Hrs.:Mins. per Wk.
1	Swim	4 (5)	8	1.9 min.	20	2:21
2	Swim	4 (5)	8	1.6 min.	20	2:11
3	Swim	4 (5)	10	1.5 min.	20	2:20
4	Swim	4 (5)	10	1.3 min.	20	2:12
5	Swim	4 (5)	12	1.8 min.	20	2:46
6	Swim	4 (5)	12	1.3 min.	20	2:22
7	Swim	4 (5)	14	1.4 min.	20	2:28
8	Swim	4 (5)	16	1.3 min.	20	2:43
9	Swim	4 (5)	18	1.3 min.	20	2:54
10	Swim	5	18	1.3 min.	20	3:37
11	Swim	4 (5)	20	1.2 min.	20	2:56
12	Swim	5	20	1.2 min.	20	3:40

*If you want to do the seven-day program in chapter 10, make sure you have your doctor's okay first. We discovered in our live-in program that weight loss was accelerated by additional daily workout sessions during the start-up period. When you are at your cardiovascular fitness level, as shown in the plan for the tenth week, you must continue to exercise a minimum of thirty minutes per day, five days per week, to make a permanent impact on your set point.
**If you want to reduce muscle soreness and prevent injury, we recommend the flexibility program in the next chapter.

PLAN II:
PERSONAL START-UP PLAN FOR SWIMMING
(Healthy, Over 35)

WEEKLY GOALS

Step	What to Do	Times per Wk.*	No. of Laps	Time per Lap	Flexibility** (mins.)	Total Hrs.:Mins. per Wk.
1	Swim	4 (5)	6	2.0 min.	20	2:08
2	Swim	4 (5)	6	1.6 min.	20	1:58
3	Swim	4 (5)	8	1.6 min.	20	2:11
4	Swim	4 (5)	8	1.5 min.	20	2:08
5	Swim	4 (5)	10	1.4 min.	20	2:16
6	Swim	4 (5)	10	1.3 min.	20	2:12
7	Swim	4 (5)	12	1.3 min.	20	2:22
8	Swim	4 (5)	14	1.4 min.	20	2:38
9	Swim	4 (5)	16	1.4 min.	20	2:50
10	Swim	4 (5)	18	1.2 min.	20	2:46
11	Swim	5	18	1.2 min.	20	3:28
12	Swim	5	20	1.2 min.	20	3:40

*If you want to do the seven-day program in chapter 10, make sure you have your doctor's okay first. We discovered in our live-in program that weight loss was accelerated by additional daily workout sessions during the start-up period. When you are at your cardiovascular fitness level, as shown in the plan for the tenth week, you must continue to exercise a minimum of thirty minutes per day, five days per week, to make a permanent impact on your set point.
**If you want to reduce muscle soreness and prevent injury, we recommend the flexibility program in the next chapter.

Once you have selected the appropriate plan, your next decision should be how often you will swim each week. Under the "Times Per Week" column on the Swimming Start-up charts, the first number is what we recommend if you are primarily concerned with aerobic fitness. The number in parentheses is the number of times to exercise if you also want to lose weight; you need to work out more frequently in order to affect your set point. In addition, both charts include the recommended number of minutes of flexibility training that should be part of your balanced workout program. So the indicated total hours and minutes per week include the amount of exercise time required for cardiovascular fitness *plus* twenty minutes a day, five days a week, for flexibility.

YOUR PERSONAL HIGH-ENERGY BIKING PROGRAM

Do you remember your first bike? Dave got his in the middle of World War II. In those days you couldn't buy a new bike or a car, so his was a used bike shared with his younger brother. Nevertheless, memories of those exciting days still provide the ambience for today's biking activities.

Bikes are even more exciting today, with the wide range of options available in equipment, tires, gears, gear ratios, accessories, and clothing. If you like gadgets, there's an endless selection.

Biking is also a good entree to social activities and sporting events. The Appalachian Mountain Club, for example, sponsors cycling tours and trips. In southern climes biking activities abound year round! When winter weather puts a damper on biking in other parts of the country, some bicycle enthusiasts put their bikes on stands and—presto!—they have an exercise machine. Of course, you can also buy a bike exerciser for those cold and windy days.

STATIONARY BIKES AS AN ALTERNATIVE TO BICYCLING

Like regular bikes, stationary cycles come in different price ranges. At the top of the line are highly sophisticated machines controlled by computers. They do practically everything but

AEROBIC FITNESS RATING FOR BIKING

Pace of Activity	Calories Burned		Aerobic Fitness Rating
	20 mins.	30 mins.	
Biking 6 mph	80	120	Low. This is for people who cannot exercise vigorously.
Biking 10 mph	120	180	Medium
Biking 11 mph	140	210	Medium
Biking 12 mph	180	270	Medium
Biking 13 mph	220	330	High

brush your teeth. If you are into gadgets and can afford it, by all means buy one. They allow you to select from a number of increasingly difficult exercise levels that include warm-ups and simulated uphill cycling. Popular state-of-the art stationary bikes can cost as much as $1,500; at the other end of the scale you can get a perfectly serviceable bike with a cast-iron wheel, a mechanical timer, odometer, speedometer, and an adjustable pressure lever for as little as $100.

ADVANTAGES OF A HIGH-ENERGY BIKING PROGRAM

- You'll experience less strain on your muscles and joints than in running. If you have knee problems, biking is preferable to walking since you don't put weight on your knees when you bike.
- Biking is fun! It brings back memories of happy childhood adventures and provides lots of fresh air.
- You can do many personal errands on your bike, rather than driving or taking public transportation.
- You can bike alone or in a group.
- You can collect and tinker with different kinds of cycles.
- There are many tours, clubs, and social groups for cross-country trips and weekend outings.

While biking has a long list of fun-filled advantages, it is easy not to work hard enough to get the proper cardiovascular fitness result. To get an aerobic fitness rating of "High," as you can see from the chart below, you must pedal at 13 miles per hour. And this has to be done continuously, so those long downhill coasts don't count. A stationary bike, of course, solves that problem.

BIKING DRAWBACKS

The disadvantages in selecting on-the-road biking as your primary energy-building cardiovascular exercise include bad weather and careless motorists. Try to use quiet streets, or stay on special paths where cars are not allowed. If you plan on doing a lot of biking, you should wear protective headgear. Maintenance is also a problem: Bikes must be kept in tip-top condition, and if you are doing any off-road biking, maintenance will need to be more frequent.

YOUR PERSONAL HIGH-ENERGY BIKING START-UP PROGRAM

Below are two start-up plans for people who are in good health. Plan I is for men and women under thirty-five, and for those who already have been exercising and want a more vigorous workout. Plan II is for those over thirty-five. Do not begin either program—even if you feel you are healthy—without the approval of your physician. If your physician believes these plans are too strenuous for you, ask for a modified plan. It is perfectly all right to start out slowly and build up to physical fitness. The important thing is that you start moving, no matter what your pace!

Once you have selected the appropriate plan, your next decision should be how often you will exercise each week. Under the "Times per Week" column on the chart, the first number is what we recommend if you are primarily concerned with aerobic fitness. The number in parentheses is the recommended number of

PLAN I:
PERSONAL START-UP PLAN FOR BIKING
(Healthy, Under 35)
WEEKLY GOALS

Step	What to Do	Times per Wk.*	Miles	Mins. per Mile	Miles per Hour	Flexibility** (Mins.)	Total Hrs.:Mins. per Wk.
1	Pedal	3	5	6	10	20	2:30
2	Pedal	3 (5)	5	5	12	20	2:15
3	Pedal	4 (5)	5	4	15	20	2:40
4	Pedal	4 (5)	6	4.5	13	20	3:08
5	Pedal	4 (5)	6	4	15	20	2:56
6	Pedal	4 (5)	7	4.5	13	20	3:26
7	Pedal	4 (5)	7	4	15	20	3:12
8	Pedal	4 (5)	8	4.5	13	20	3:44
9	Pedal	4 (5)	8	4.3	14	20	3:38
10	Pedal	4 (5)	8	4	15	20	3:28

*If you want to do the seven-day program in chapter 10, make sure you have your doctor's okay first. We discovered in our live-in program that weight loss was accelerated by additional daily workout sessions during the start-up period. When you are at your cardiovascular fitness level, as shown in the plan for the tenth week, you must continue to exercise a minimum of thirty minutes per day, five days per week, to make a permanent impact on your set point.

**If you want to reduce muscle soreness and prevent injury, we recommend the flexibility program in the next chapter.

times to exercise if you also want to lose weight. To do that you need to work out more frequently in order to affect your set point. Both charts also include the recommended number of minutes of flexibility training that should be part of your balanced workout program. So the indicated total hours and minutes per week include the amount of exercise time required for cardiovascular fitness, *plus* twenty minutes a day, five days a week, for flexibility.

Both programs peak at the same point: eight miles a day at 15 miles per hour (four-minute miles). If this is not strenuous enough for you, you can either speed up a bit or add a mile to the distance. *Use your common sense and listen to your body.* Unless you fall or get hit by a car, it's pretty hard to hurt yourself by pedaling.

PLAN II:
PERSONAL START-UP PLAN FOR BIKING
(Healthy, Over 35)
WEEKLY GOALS

Step	What to Do	Times per Wk.*	Miles	Mins. per Mile	Miles per Hour	Flexibility** (Mins.)	Total Hrs.:Mins. per Wk.
1	Pedal	3 (5)	4	6	10	20	2:12
2	Pedal	3 (5)	4	5	12	20	2:00
3	Pedal	4 (5)	5	6	10	20	3:20
4	Pedal	4 (5)	5	5	12	20	3:00
5	Pedal	4 (5)	5	4.5	13	20	2:50
6	Pedal	4 (5)	6	4.3	14	20	3:03
7	Pedal	4 (5)	6	4	15	20	2:56
8	Pedal	4 (5)	7	4.5	13	20	3:26
9	Pedal	4 (5)	7	4.3	14	20	3:20
10	Pedal***	4 (5)	7	4	15	20	3:12
11	Pedal	4 (5)	8	4.2	14	20	3:34
12	Pedal	4 (5)	8	4	15	20	3:28

*If you want to do the seven-day program in chapter 10, make sure you have your doctor's okay first. We discovered in our live-in program that weight loss was acccelerated by additional daily workout sessions during the start-up period. When you are at your cardiovascular fitness level, as shown in the plan for the tenth week, you must continue to exercise a minimum of thirty minutes per day, five days per week, to make a permanent impact on your set point. (You can get by with twenty minutes on a stationary bike.)

**If you want to reduce muscle soreness and help prevent injury, we recommend the flexibility program in the next chapter.

***Acceptable cardiovascular fitness can be maintained here at step 10.

A HIGH-ENERGY RUNNING/JOGGING PROGRAM

Many running aficionados like to make distinctions between running and jogging. Jogging has been defined as bouncing up and down as you move at a walking pace. Others say you are running only when you can make a mile in less than nine minutes. For people into competitive sports, these distinctions are probably important. For people interested in maintaining a high level of energy and fitness, they are irrelevant. What is important is that you jog or run fast enough and long enough to get your heart beat up to 70 to 80 percent of its capacity and keep it there for fifteen minutes. We've decided to combine jogging and running into one category. Regardless of what you call this activity, its advantages are substantial.

AEROBIC FITNESS RATINGS FOR RUNNING/JOGGING

Pace of Activity	Calories Burned		Aerobic Fitness Rating
	20 mins.	30 mins.	
Running/Jogging 1 mile in 12 min.	160	240	High
Running/Jogging 1 mile in 11 min.	200	300	High
Running/Jogging 1 mile in 10 min.	220	330	High

CONSIDERATIONS ON RUNNING/JOGGING

If you decide you want to run or jog, to avoid injury it is essential that you warm up properly. Recent research indicates that inappropriate warm-up exercises can themselves cause injury and that a moderate cooling down phase is more effective in guarding against injuries. This is because people tend to "snap" muscles in warm-up exercises by stretching them to the extreme, rapidly and repeatedly tensing and untensing them. If your muscles aren't warmed up to begin with, this snapping action can cause injury.

A few minutes of walking is the best warm-up for running or jogging. Or if you're in pretty good shape, run or jog at a slower than normal pace for a few minutes. Then after your run, cool down by walking for at least another five minutes.

Our exercise route is three miles, but we run only two of them. We walk for a few minutes from our house to the start of our "course." Then we run for twenty minutes. By this time we have covered about two and a quarter miles, counting both the walking and running. Then we walk home for approximately three-quarters of a mile. It works out well.

Another drawback to running is the pounding your body takes. While this pounding helps to strengthen bones, it can have a negative effect on joints. Good running shoes go a long way toward minimizing the problem. Many athletic clubs have padded tracks. Running or jogging on dirt or grass is easier on the joints than pavement, but you have to watch out for such impediments as holes or uneven ground.

Stretching Out Shin Splints
Note from Joely

Our stretching routine has solved shin splint problems for a number of our Never Be Tired Again graduates. Shin splints are painful microscopic tears in the muscles of your shins.

Sandy owns Bunty Lee Stables, a riding academy in Londonderry, New Hampshire. She took up running as a way to help reduce stress. Running a riding academy may not at first glance seem like a stressful job. After all, she is outdoors a lot; horses don't talk back or tell you that the head office just cut your budget and increased your work load at the same time. However, if you knew how much she has to pay for liability insurance you'd begin to understand the stress Sandy faces.

When Sandy entered our program she had not been able to run for months because of shin splints. We put her on our flexibility program (described in the next chapter), and in just one week she was back running without pain. A year later, Sandy is still doing the flexibility stretches, still running, and even has added biking to her exercise regimen. All this with no recurrence of her shin splint problem!

You need not wait until you have an injury to benefit from the flexibility program. It's a wonderful way to counteract the muscle-tightening effect of aerobic exercise. We experienced that ourselves five years ago when we decided to add running to our personal exercise program as an alternative when we traveled and couldn't find a pool. Until then swimming had been our primary cardiovascular exercise, coupled with a modest yoga routine.

Bright and early one morning, David took his first distance run in thirty years by running a mile and a half and walking a mile and a half. Since he was already cardiovascularly fit from our swimming program, his main concern was sore muscles. Guess what? No sore muscles. Apparently the years of yoga-style stretching did the trick. The next day David ran three miles. Since then running has become one of his two primary exercise programs. (Fast walking is the other.) Later on, I decided to join him in it. Because of my stretching program, I had only minor soreness in my Achilles tendons the first week—a small miracle for someone who has worn high heels every day of her adult life.

MINIMIZING THE RISK OF INJURY: THE ALEXANDER TECHNIQUE

Another effective way to minimize the risk of injury and simultaneously improve performance is to learn how to use your body more efficiently and with greater ease. An excellent method for achieving those two goals is the Alexander Technique. We have recently applied it to our normal activities. While the technique has broader applications than its use in cardiovascular exercise, we feel this is an appropriate time to introduce it because of its ability to reduce the risk of injury during vigorous physical activities.

More than twenty-five years of research, much of it conducted at Tufts University Institute for Experimental Psychology, plus an enormous amount of accumulated clinical information provide substantial evidence that the technique helps people

- Learn to release chronic physical tensions
- Improve spinal alignment and posture
- Improve muscular coordination
- Improve muscle tone
- Get rid of unconscious but unwanted muscle responses to physical and emotional stimuli and substitute healthier ones

If you ask someone who has taken Alexander lessons to describe the experience, he or she would be hard-pressed to put it into words. That's because the Alexander Technique has to be experienced to be fully understood.

The technique was developed at the turn of the century by F. Matthias Alexander, an Australian actor who kept losing his voice. Unable to get help from conventional sources, Alexander began to study himself with mirrors. He found that when he began to speak in public he put downward pressure on his spine by moving his head backward and downward. He developed a method to stop himself from doing this. In the process, he discovered the enormous potential of learning to "use the self," as he called it, in a different and more effective way. Eventually this led to the Alexander Technique, an organized method for controlling undesirable physical reactions and substituting more appropriate ones.

While few people have been able to learn the Alexander Technique on their own, the beauty of the system is that the goal of the instruction is to show you how to carry it out yourself.

Many prominent people have been proponents of the technique, including Aldous Huxley, George Bernard Shaw, and John Dewey. Dewey, the famous educational philosopher, began his lessons at age fifty-eight. He atrributed much of the rejuvenation and vigor of the next thirty-five years of his life to the technique.

In spite of the research, the clinical data, and the testimony of those who have used it, the Alexander Technique has until recently been a well-kept secret in the United States. We recommend that anyone who exercises vigorously consider taking Alexander Technique lessons to help improve the ability to move freely under stress and thus minimize the risk of injury. This technique has made it possible for us to gain greater benefits from our flexibility training. As we progress, we find that it helps us with our visualizations, too.

You can find out about Alexander Technique teachers in your area by contacting the Alexander Technique Association of New England (15A Channing Street, Cambridge, MA 02138; 617-497-2242) or the American Center for the Alexander Technique (142 West End Avenue, New York, NY 10023; 212-799-0468).

YOUR PERSONAL HIGH-ENERGY RUNNING/ JOGGING START-UP PLAN

Below are two start-up plans for those in good health. Plan I is for men and women under thirty-five, and for those who already have been exercising and want a more vigorous workout. Plan II is for those over thirty-five. Do not follow either of these programs (even if you are healthy) without the approval of your physician. If your physician feels the plan is too strenuous for your present physical condition, ask for a modified plan. It's okay to start out slowly and build up to physical fitness. The important thing is that you start moving, no matter what the pace!

Once you have chosen the appropriate plan, your next decision should be how often you will exercise each week. Under the "Times per Week" column on the chart, the first number is what we suggest if you are primarily concerned with aerobic fitness. The number in parentheses is the recommended number of times to exercise if you also want to lose weight. In order to affect your set point, you'll need to work out more frequently. In addition, both charts include the recommended number of minutes of flexibility training that should be part of your balanced workout program. So the indicated hours and minutes per week include the amount of exercise time required for cardiovascular fitness, *plus* twenty minutes a day, five days a week, for flexibility.

PLAN I:
PERSONAL START-UP PLAN FOR RUNNING/JOGGING
(Healthy, Under 35)

WEEKLY GOALS

Step	What to Do	Times per Wk.*	Miles	Minutes per Mile	Cool Down (Mins.)	Flexibility** (Mins.)	Total Hrs.:Mins. per Wk.
1	Walk	3 (5)	2.0	15	n/a	20	2:30
2	Walk	3 (5)	3.0	15	n/a	20	3:15
3	Walk/ run	4 (5)	2.0	13	5	20	3:24
4	Walk/ run	4 (5)	2.0	12	5	20	3:16
5	Run	4 (5)	2.0	11	5	20	3:08
6	Run	4 (5)	2.0	10	5	20	3:00
7	Run	5	2.0	10	5	20	3:45
8	Run	4 (5)	2.5	10	5	20	3:20
9	Run	4 (5)	2.5	9.5	5	20	3:15
10	Run	4 (5)	3.0	9	5	20	3:28

*If you want to do the seven-day program in chapter 10, make sure you have your doctor's okay first. We discovered in our live-in program that weight loss was accelerated by additional workout sessions during the start-up period. When you are at your cardiovascular fitness level, as shown in the plan for the tenth week, you must continue to run a minimum of twenty minutes per day, five days per week, to make a permanent impact on your set point.
**If you want to reduce muscle soreness and prevent injury, we recommend the flexibility program in the next chapter.

PLAN II:
PERSONAL START-UP PLAN FOR RUNNING/JOGGING
(Healthy, Over 35)
WEEKLY GOALS

Step	What to Do	Times per Wk.*	Miles	Minutes per Mile	Cool Down (Mins.)	Flexibility** (Mins.)	Total Hrs.:Mins. per Wk.
1	Walk	3 (5)	2.0	17	0	20	2:24
2	Walk	3 (5)	2.5	17	0	20	3:08
3	Walk	3 (5)	3.0	16.5	0	20	3:29
4	Walk/ run	4 (5)	2.0	13	5	20	3:24
5	Walk/ run	4 (5)	2.0	12	5	20	3:16
6	Run	4 (5)	2.0	11	5	20	3:08
7	Run	4 (5)	2.0	10	5	20	3:00
8	Run	5	2.0	10	5	20	3:45
9	Run	4 (5)	2.5	10	5	20	3:20
10	Run	4 (5)	3.0	10	5	20	3:40

*If you want to do the seven-day program in chapter 10, make sure you have your doctor's okay first. We discovered in our live-in program that weight loss was accelerated by additional workout sessions during the start-up period. When you are at your cardiovascular fitness level, as shown in the plan for the tenth week, you must continue to run a minimum of twenty minutes per day, five days per week, to make a permanent impact on your set point.
**If you want to reduce muscle soreness and prevent injury, we recommend the flexibility program in the next chapter.

CROSS-COUNTRY SKIING AS A HIGH-ENERGY OPTION

An hour of cross-country skiing is an excellent substitute for *any* cardiovascular exercise. You don't need a chart to know how great a workout you're getting! In addition to your legs, you use your upper body and arms to push with the poles. Cross-country skiing is fun for all the family and offers all the social advantages of downhill skiing, without the latter's hazards.

ADVANTAGES OF AN ENERGY-BUILDING CROSS-COUNTRY SKIING OPTION

- It provides more aerobic benefits than running because more of your muscles are involved.

- It's easier to learn than downhill skiing.
- You can do it by yourself or with friends and family.
- You can join organized groups that sponsor skiing weekends and tours.
- You can make it a competitive sport if you wish.

HOW FAST? HOW FAR?

People who are just starting to exercise usually ask the same two questions. How fast should I go? How far should I go? There is no "right" answer to those questions. How fast you should go depends entirely on what shape you're in. You need to go fast enough to maintain an energy-building heart rate of 70 to 80 percent of your maximum heart rate. Please don't think that by exceeding your EBHR you will gain greater benefits. This is *not* a case where if some is good, more is better. When your heart rate is between 70 and 80 percent of its capacity, your body burns more fat than blood sugar.

Instead of asking how far you should go, you should ask about the time involved. Remember that you need to be at your energy-building heart rate for at least fifteen minutes, and you need five minutes or more to build up to that rate. So the absolute minimum amount of time you should give to the exercise is twenty minutes (thirty minutes if you're walking). The good news is that your body gets approximately two-thirds of its energy by burning fat during the first half hour of aerobic exercise.

QUICK ENERGY CHARGE #14

Five-Minute Preworkout Battery Charge
Step 1: Getting ready to charge your battery
Put on your workout clothes so you will be ready to go as soon as your five-minute "battery charge" is completed. (If you want to take more time to get "charged," it's okay.) You can do this exercise at home or at a spot near where you plan to start your workout (for example, at a bench near the pool or a wall near where you begin your fast walk).

Step 2: Mind set
Close your eyes and breathe in through your nose very slowly and

deeply. Fill your stomach first, then your midriff, and then your upper chest. You may want to raise your shoulders slightly to allow even more oxygen to enter your lungs. Hold this breath for a count of four, then exhale slowly through your mouth. As you exhale, feel your shoulders relax and drop and the muscles in your upper body become less tense and cramped. Say to yourself, "It is all right to give myself this time each day. It is essential that I recharge myself. The more oxygen I can generate, the more healthy, vital, and productive I feel."

Step 3. Counting down

Keeping your eyes closed, take a deep breath and exhale slowly. With your mind's eye, scan every muscle in your body. Notice that you are a bit more relaxed than you were before you took that first deep breath. Next, with each long slow breath, begin counting down from 5 to 1. Inhale as you say "five," exhale as you say "five" again and imagine yourself going down a flight of stairs. Continue counting down through 1. Notice that with each breath and each stair you are more relaxed than you were before.

After you have taken the five breaths and are at the bottom of the stairs, see yourself walking through a beautiful forest—lush, green, warm, inviting. Walk toward a crystal-clear pond and lie on the soft grass next to it. See yourself completely alone, secure, and totally relaxed. Feel the sun shining on you, keeping you snug and warm.

Step 4: Deepening your memory

Pay attention to what it feels like to be alert and relaxed at the same time. Say to yourself, "Each time I count from five to one, I reach a more profound, relaxed, and creative level of mind than the last time I entered this level of consciousness."

Step 5: Sensing your internal energy

Now, breathing normally, pay attention to the sound and sensations of your body. Remember that your body, as an energy system, is made up of a large network of vibrating strings of energy. Allow those strings to vibrate in harmony with one another. Feel the oneness that comes from this recognition. If other thoughts come into your mind, pretend you are simply an observer of your body. Let those thoughts pass through your head without judgment. Continue to focus on the vibrations of your energy strings.

Step 6: Energy programming
Breathing slowly and deeply, see the oxygen entering every cell in your body. See your tiredness and tension melting into the floor, leaving you relaxed and alert. With each breath, breathe in increased energy and breathe out tiredness and stress. See the energy come into your body as pure white light.

Now that your deepest self is tuned in and harmonizing in this relaxed but alert state, form a mental picture of yourself exercising effortlessly and joyously. Say to yourself as you inhale, "I am growing," and as you exhale, "stronger and healthier every day in every way." Continue to repeat this battery-charging breathing exercise until your inner voice tells you it is time to begin your cardiovascular exercise program.

Step7: Reentry: The final charge
Say to yourself, "I am bursting with energy." Sense yourself harmonizing with all the vibrating energy strings of the creative force. Know that you are connected in oneness with the infinite network of energy that is the universe and that you always can have an abundance of this energy just by exercising. Say to yourself, "My body is ready to accept all of the energy that I need from the universe as I (run, swim, walk, bike)." Now listen to your breathing. When you are ready, open your eyes, stretch, and go about your daily exercise joyously, knowing you are increasing your energy, feeling better than you did before.

QUICK ENERGY CHARGE #15

High-Energy Awareness: Boosting Your Workout
Mind set
As you begin to exercise, say to yourself, "When I exercise, I enter a state of total awareness where I generate an endless stream of high-energy molecules."

Focusing
To become focused, repeat the following phrase silently or aloud: "I am in complete control of my body." Say this over and over

until you can sense that your muscles are warmed up (about five minutes).

Note: You do not have to use these particular words. You can use any phrase you want as long as you keep it short. The point is to center your attention on your physical activity in the focused manner of a mindfulness procedure. We use different phrases just for variety, such as "I'm growing stronger and more powerful with each stroke (step, stride)."

Body scan

Once you are focused and your muscles are warm, begin using your mind's "flashlight" to scan every muscle, joint, and bone in your body. Notice the sensations in your toes, the balls of your feet, ankles, calves, thighs, etc. Review every inch of your body right up to the top of your head. Note every sensation. At the end of the body scan, try to feel all the combined physical sensations that your body receives as you exercise. Note all the sensations, but do not judge them.

Total environment scan

Now focus your attention on the sounds, smells, and sights around you as you move through or in your exercise environment. If you are swimming, notice the sensations you feel from the moisture on your skin as you glide through the water. If you are walking, running, or biking, inhale and smell and taste the air that surrounds you. Hear every sound, see every sight, feel every sensation. Remember, the goal of this exercise is to be open and focused enough to be completely aware of everyting in your environment, including your own body and mind, all at once. Focus simultaneously on feelings, sounds, tactile sensations, and thoughts. Let judgments about these sensations or thoughts pass through your mind like puffy white clouds.

Muscle and joint tune-up

Notice that as you enter this state of total awareness your exercise movements become easier. You are fast-walking (jogging, swimming, biking) effortlessly. Now take your mind's flashlight and shine your internal light on your toes. Say to yourself, "My toes are in tune with the energy vibrations of my entire body." Sense the fine tuning of the energy vibrations in your toes as if you were a mechanic tuning a race car engine. Notice the subtle and pleasant difference in how your toes feel as you tune their energy vibrations while in motion. Repeat the process for the balls of your feet, the whole foot, your ankles, your calves, your shins, your knees, and so on until you reach the top of your head.

Energy charge

Now that your body and mind are totally aware and finely tuned, use your mind's flashlight to illuminate each and every cell in your body. Say to yourself, "With every stride (stroke, step) my cells are creating more and more high-energy molecules (ATP) in a never ending stream. I'm getting stronger and healthier with every moment that I exercise." Sense the subtle difference in your energy level as the vision of your own internal energy manufacturing process gets more and more efficient. Say to yourself, "I feel wonderful every time I exercise!"

Options

To get the maximum benefits of this mindfulness technique, it is not necessary to complete all of the sections we have listed each time you exercise. But you must begin each session with "Mind Set," following with the "Focusing" session. After that, you can choose to do just the "Body Scan" or the "Total Environment Scan" or the "Muscle and Joint Scan"—or any combination thereof. However, please end each session with the "Energy Charge."

Chapter 21

Stretch for
High Energy

What happens to the flexibility and energy we all are born with? Must we accept that they disappear over time?

Absolutely not!

ENERGY, FLEXIBILITY, AND OXYGEN

Even though regular cardiovascular exercise will help you build up energy by increasing your ATP production, it will not increase or even maintain flexibility.

It is a physiological fact that muscles shorten and contract as your body moves. A contracted muscle cannot absorb blood. Since blood carries oxygen, this means that during exercise the muscles are not getting as much oxygen. Stretching, which lengthens muscles, allows for improved blood flow. Poor circulation, on the other hand, can cause muscle pain, which causes more contraction, which causes further pain—its a vicious circle.

Joints are also affected by muscles that are too tight. A joint—whether the knee, the elbow, the wrist—surrounded by contracted muscles does not have the full range of motion it was meant to have. The body, amazing structure that it is, compensates by making some other joint do more work. But this adjustment pulls the body out of alignment, further compounding stiffness problems.

The good news is that you can regain flexibility at any age by stretching.

THE FIVE GOALS OF YOUR STRETCHING PROGRAM

1. Get more oxygenated blood into your muscles to create more energy. You also will heal and nourish muscles that might otherwise be strained or damaged by your cardiovascular exercise program.
2. Become more agile, flexibile, and toned.
3. Learn to relax your muscles completely at will, letting your mind and body benefit from the profound easing of strain.
4. Learn to stimulate your glands and internal organs in such a way that they function more efficiently. This includes helping your system to better eliminate the toxic by-products of your digestive process.
5. Learn to control your breathing for better physical performance.

YOGA: A PROVEN, AGE-OLD PROGRAM FOR FLEXIBILITY

Yoga, the stretching program we recommend, is the oldest physical program of its kind. A major goal of this program is to break the vicious circle that begins when you become less active and, as a result, your spine stiffens up.

A stretching program is *not* calisthenics.

If you have ever done any kind of calisthenics, we're sure you will notice the similarity of yoga positions to some exercises. It is only a fleeting similarity, however, because yoga poses are far superior in their ability to improve flexibility, to reduce tension, and to increase the flow of oxygenated blood to the muscles. Calisthenics emphasize quick, jerking movements that "snap" the muscles. The major emphasis is on motion. In yoga there is a negative emphasis on motion. The postions are called *poses* for a reason, and the reason is that yoga emphasizes holding muscles in a gentle stretch followed by a gentle release.

Imagine a rubber band: In calisthenics the goal is to pull the band out and snap it back quickly; in yoga, the goal is to stretch the rubber band slowly, hold it stretched, and then release it gently. The muscles and spinal column get an excellent workout without the risk of injury inherent in calisthenics.

THE BENEFITS OF A STRETCHING PROGRAM BASED ON YOGA

Physical Benefits	Psychological Benefits
More resilient muscles	
Taut skin	A sense of inner peace
Increased energy and vitality	Quieter mind
Increased suppleness and flexibility	Ability to relax completely at will
Improved complexion and a more youthful appearance	Relief of tension
	Improved self-concept
Stronger and cleaner lungs	Better sleep
Normal bowels	
Normal weight	
Trim body, improved circulation	

There are few if any risks in doing yoga. Our program involves gentle stretching movements and the holding of poses while concentrating on breathing and relaxation. Yoga flexibility and stretching exercises should be done slowly and gently.

Caution: If you have any physical problems or injuries, get your physician's approval before beginning your yoga stretches.

SIX THOUSAND YEARS OF EXPERIENCE

Anyone from any religion (or no religion) can adopt the science of yoga. It is a time-tested method with more than 6,000 years of experience in self-development programming! The branch of yoga that concerns us—hatha yoga—is the world's oldest known physical culture. In recent years Western scientists and physicians have studied hatha yoga with modern equipment and techniques. Their findings increasingly show that the practice of yoga makes profound physiological and psychological changes in human beings.

Joely's Yoga Story

My first experience with yoga took place sixteen years ago when I took a yoga course at a local YWCA. I enjoyed the course, though I was somewhat discouraged to find I wasn't nearly as flexible as I thought I'd be. I'd always been a fairly active child, and I was a cheerleader in high school, doing all the jumping and tumbling involved in that. It never occurred to me that my body might be tightening up and losing the flexibility I assumed would always be there, sort of as my God-given gift.

It was a rude awakening to find I couldn't manage even some of the "simple" bending and stretching positions as well as I thought I should be able to. The real killer was the leg-stretch pose (pictured later in this chapter). In this pose you sit on the floor, bend forward, and stretch so that you rest your head on your knees. I could no more get my head anywhere near my knees than I could fly. I was lucky if I could bend forward a third of the way—and I was still in my early twenties and considered myself in good shape.

Insult was added to injury when I noticed a woman in her fifties who was able to put her forehead flat to her knees as if she were hinged at the hips. I made a point of speaking to the woman during class. She told me she had been studying yoga for a few years. She assured me, however, that when she began yoga classes she was in no better shape than I was then.

About ten years ago, under David's influence, I went back to yoga. At the same time I changed my eating habits to more closely resemble the diet we describe in the section on nutrition (chapters 7 through 13). Because I was trying to combat feelings of extreme tiredness in mid-morning and mid-afternoon, I ate small amounts of the right food six times a day. I had fruit or nonfat yogurt around 10:30 A.M. and 3:30 P.M. and had another snack in the evening after dinner. David would set an alarm to remind me to eat, because it was getting to a point where I was rebelling against snacking all the time. All I could think of was, "Oh, no, I have to eat again."

Within two months of practicing yoga and improving my diet, I experienced a great boost in vitality. Although I had not changed my diet to lose weight, my clothes now hung loosely on me. I had lost about ten pounds without really trying. I attribute both the increased energy and the decreased weight to the interaction of yoga and diet. Without knowing it, I had begun to implement part of the Never Be Tired Again program! And I am now more flexible than I was seventeen years ago.

Breathing is the key to oxygen flow.

The word *hatha* is made up of two Sanskrit roots, *ha* and *tha*. *Ha* literally means "sun" but is interpreted to mean the flow of the breath through the right nostril. Similarly, *tha* means "moon" but is interpreted to mean the flow of the breath through the left nostril. Thus *hatha yoga* means "union of the two breaths." Physical or hatha yoga emphasizes breath control when stretching, moving, or meditating. As you will see, breath control is a fundamental part of the stretching program outlined in this chapter. It is the key to getting more oxygen into your lungs while at the same time helping to relax your muscles so that the oxygenated blood can flow more readily into every part of your body.

THE IMPORTANCE OF THE MIND-BODY LINK

What you visualize before and during the stretching movements is just as important as what you do when you move your body. Your aim is to gain mental control over your physical being. Part of the secret is breath control, part is the use of visualization techniques that enhance performance. Modern sports medicine recognizes the value of this approach. For example, many Olympic champions are trained to visualize what they are going to do just prior to doing it. They also are trained to use breath control as an aid to smooth physical functioning. The ultimate reality is that there is no true separation of mind and body.

ELEVEN WAYS TO ENSURE A SUCCESSFUL STRETCHING WORKOUT

Follow these psychologically and physically oriented suggestions for improving your performance and progress in our stretching program.

1. Pay attention to atmosphere. Find a quiet, private place. Since comfort is an important part of the atmosphere around you, it helps to work out on a padded rug or exercise mat. Many positions can be uncomfortable if performed on a hard surface.

2. Set reasonable goals. Measurable goals in yoga are different from measurable goals in calisthenics. Rather than being concerned with how many times or how quickly you can do a specific pose, your goal should be to see how *slowly* you can perform a movement. Here's another goal: to be totally present while doing your yoga, as opposed to going through the physical motions but being mentally miles away. Unreasonable goals can easily lead to pulled muscles.

3. Give yourself plenty of room. In picking your yoga location, make sure you have enough space so you can stretch out on all four sides. Move any furniture that might be in the way.

4. Wear loose clothing. For private sessions, men find bikini-type briefs comfortable; women may prefer to go without a bra if it tends to bind. When doing yoga in group sessions, running shorts and T-shirts or leotards are usually the best choice. Make sure your shorts have an elasticized waistband; you don't want anything cutting into you.

5. *More is better.* Your stretching program should be done four to five times a week. Flexibility training is one regimen where a little is good and more is better. If you can make the program a regular part of your schedule, try doing it every day.

6. *Coordinate with your cardiovascular exercise program.* If you choose running or biking as your daily exercise, you should do your stretching program *after* you exercise. The reason? Running tightens your muscles; yoga stretches them out again and releases the lactic acid buildup. Swimming is not as tightening, so you can alternate your stretching and swimming programs if you wish. Of course, in order to have a cardiovascular and a stretching workout four to five times a week, there will be overlap days when you will need to do both. At any rate, you will feel more psychologically relaxed if you follow your cardiovascular workout with gentle stretching, breathing, and visualization.

7. *Don't do stretching movements on a full stomach.* Wait at least two hours after eating, or do them before breakfast. Since many of the movements and postures are designed to massage internal organs, this can interfere with your digestion if your stomach is full.

8. *Treat yourself gently.* The movements and postures in our stretching program are not exercises. Understanding this basic concept is essential to successful performance. You should *not* be tired at the end of a stretching session; rather, you should feel rested and relaxed. If your muscles are sore, you are not stretching correctly. The idea is to stretch as far as you can without pain and then hold. If you go too far or too quickly, you will hurt yourself.

9. *Take your time.* Progress never comes in a straight line. Some days you'll make more progress than others. Just take it easy; relax and let your body respond over time. One of the great things about this program is that you can start at any age and expect to make progress. There are programs specifically designed for senior citizens that would put a twenty-year-old to shame. Look at some of the articles in *Yoga Journal* or at some of the how-to yoga books, and you'll see pictures of people in their seventies and eighties—men and women who have been doing

yoga for only a few years—standing on their heads or twisted like corkscrews, and generally acting as if they had much younger bodies (which they do).

10. Don't get competitive. Be noncompetitive with yourself and with others. If you approach this program in a competitive spirit, it won't work. Your stretching program is a time to "let go" as much as it is a time to control; it is a time to listen to your body and your breathing. In your stretching program it is important to concentrate fully on what you are doing at any given *present* moment and not to live for the future. Do the best you can at what you are doing at the moment you are doing it. Don't worry about yesterday or tomorrow, or about how well another person is doing.

11. Reward yourself. Rewards are an essential part of any program to modify your behavior permanently. Rewards need not be material ones. Psychological rewards usually work better in the long run. One of the approaches we use is to find a reward that requires us to apply our newly developed flexibility in a physical activity. Dave found great satisfaction in being able to run again after a long layoff without having a sore muscle from day one, thanks to his flexibility training.

We will be leading you through nine key stretching exercises: three warm-up exercises and six basic stretching poses. To guide you in the proper positions and movements we have illustrated the nine exercises with thirty-eight sketches.

WARM-UP MOVEMENTS AND POSITIONS

The drawings in this section will guide you in detail through the three important warm-up movements and positions: Chest Expansion, Knees to Chest, and Hands to Floor. These stretches should precede all other movements (but also may be done any time to relieve tension).

The warm-up movements help to relieve flatulence, indigestion, and tension in the chest. Joggers, runners, and walkers will find they also help ease leg and back tension.

Caution: In order not to injure yourself, yoga flexibility and stretching exercises should be done slowly and gently. If you have any physical problems or injuries, get your physician's approval before beginning.

WARM-UP: HANDS TO FLOOR

Step 1. Stand straight, hands at your side. Keeping your arms straight, slowly raise them in front of you and up towards the ceiling. When your arms are about shoulder high, inhale and begin to bend backwards as far as you comfortably can. Continue to raise your arms to the ceiling and bend backwards, but do not strain yourself.

Breathing. Inhale slowly as you bend backwards.

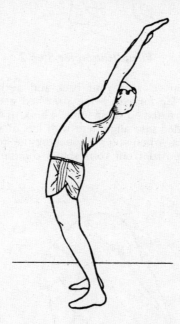

Step 2. Keep your arms straight. Exhale as you bend forward at the waist until you can touch the floor, or until you have gone as far as you can comfortably go. Try to keep your knees straight, but don't strain your lower back. Breathe normally as you hold for a count of eight.

Breathing. Exhale as you bend forward and hold.

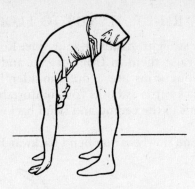

Visualization for Step 2

Concentrate on relaxing your back and neck. Create a visual picture of your leg muscles being stretched gently like a rubber band, slowly stretched to their limit. Think of your vertebrae as being gently pulled into alignment with lots of space around and between the discs. When you are touching the floor, think of your head as being loosed from your spinal column and dangling in space.

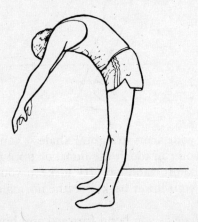

Step 3. Inhale as you slowly curl up to a standing position. *Breathing.* Slowly exhale as you relax.

Visualization for Step 3

In this step, don't just straighten up as you would in calisthenics. See your spinal column slowly rolling up like the top part of a roll-top desk, one vertebrae at a time. See the rubber band in your legs being released ever so slowly and gently.

ADDITIONAL BENEFITS OF THE HAND-TO-FLOOR POSE

In addition to relieving back and leg tension, this pose helps to

- Massage the abdominal organs, thereby relieving indigestion and constipation
- Tone the liver, kidneys, and pancreas
- Counteract menstrual disorders
- Aid in weight loss
- Trim the waist
- Firm the legs
- Invigorate the tissues of your face

WARM-UP: CHEST EXPANSION

This stretching movement is one of the best relaxation techniques we know. We do it as a way to unwind when working at the computer—about every half hour when things are tense!

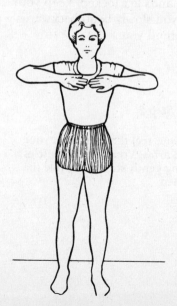

Step 1. Stand straight with your arms at your side. Bend your elbows and raise your arms so that the back of your hands touch your chest and your palms face out. *Breathing.* Inhale.

Body Focus for Step 1

Focus on relaxing your neck and lower back while you expand your chest. Feel the tension between your shoulder blades as you bring your arms up to your chest.

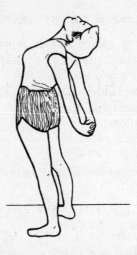

Step 2. Bring your arms around in back of you and clasp your hands behind your back. Once your hands are locked, keep your elbows straight. Hold your breath as you slowly bend backwards. Keep your arms as high as possible behind you.

Breathing. Hold your breath.

Visualization for Step 2

As you bring your arms in back of you, feel the tension in your entire upper back, shoulders, chest and arms. Visualize the muscles across your chest and in your arms being gently stretched while the muscles in your back are being contracted.

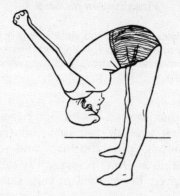

Step 3. Exhale as you slowly bend forward from the waist until your head is as close to your knees as you can bring it. Keep your arms straight and your hands locked. Now raise your hands over your head as far as you can. Breathe normally as you hold the position for a count of eight.

Visualization for Step 3

As you bend forward, relax the muscles in your neck and lead with your head. Imagine the rubber bands in your legs being stretched gently to their limit. Feel the tension in your shoulders and across your chest as your arms are stretched. Remember to "release" your neck from your shoulders and let it hang free when you are as far forward as you can go.

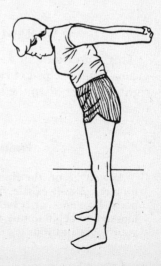

Step 4. Inhale as you slowly curl back up, keeping your hands locked and your arms straight. When you are standing, gently release your clasped hands.

Breathing. Exhale and relax.

Visualization for Step 4

Visualize your back as a roll-top desk being opened, rolling up one vertebrae at a time. As you roll up, feel the tension melting out of your neck, shoulders, and chest. Feel the rubber bands in your legs releasing gently.

Note: Don't be discouraged if you don't look exactly like the illustrations the first time or two that you try this pose. It is excellent for promoting spinal flexibility, and you will improve a little each time you do it. Don't resort to the calisthenic "bounce" to increase your range. Remember, in yoga slow and steady wins the race.

ADDITIONAL BENEFITS OF THE CHEST-EXPANSION POSE

In addition to relieving back, chest, and leg tension, this pose helps to
- Develop the bust or chest, which makes it an excellent workout companion for those who choose running as their aerobic exercise (particularly women)
- Firm the upper arms
- Expand the lungs and stimulate the lung cells
- Increase blood flow to the brain and improve mental functioning

WARM-UP: KNEES TO CHIN

This is an excellent warm-up movement for your aerobic program. It also helps get rid of indigestion and flatulence. Do your right side first, then the left, and finish with both legs at the same time.

Visualization Before Step 1

As you lie on the floor, take a deep breath and hold it for a moment. Slowly exhale, feeling the tension start to melt out of your body. Take another breath, release it slowly and feel your shoulders loosen and begin to sink into the floor. With your third breath, feel your spine and your leg muscles relax.

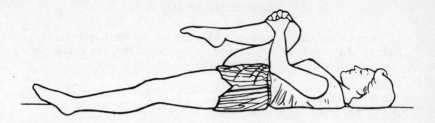

Step 1. Lie on the floor and relax. Bring your right knee to your chest. Use both hands to pull your knee down against your chest. Hold for a count of eight.

Breathing. Inhale as you bring your knee to your chest.

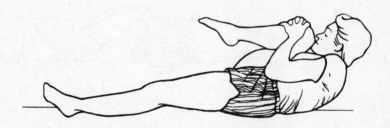

Step 2. Continue to hold your knee to your chest. Exhale as you raise your head. Curl forward and bring your chin to your knee. Hold for a count of eight.

Breathing. Exhale.

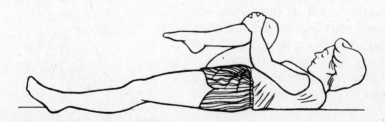

Step 3. Continue holding your knee to your chest and very slowly curl back until your head is touching the floor again.

Breathing. Breathe normally.

Visualization for Step 3

Imagine once again that your back is a roll-top desk and you are rolling the vertebrae one by one to the floor. Feel the vertebrae being gently pulled into alignment as you roll back.

Step 4. Straighten your leg, raise it vertically, and point your toes in the air.

Breathing. Inhale as you raise your leg.

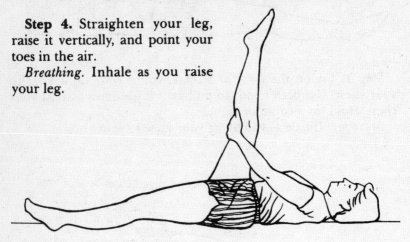

Step 5. Reach up and grasp your leg at the ankle. Exhale as you touch your chin to your knee. Breathe normally as you hold for a count of eight.

Note: In the beginning, grasp your leg wherever you can comfortably reach. If this means you grasp your leg behind the knee, that's fine. Bring your head *as close to your leg as you can manage.*

Breathing. Exhale as you bring your chin to your knee.

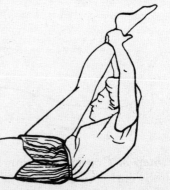

Step 6. Let go of your leg but keep it in the air while you slowly roll back to the floor.

Breathing. Breathe normally.

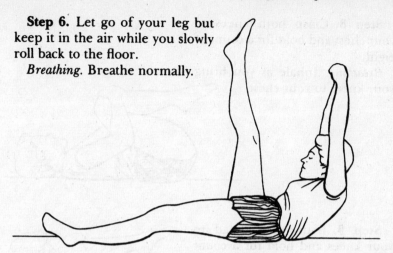

Step 7. Place your palms against the floor for added support. Slowly lower your leg to the floor to a count of eight. (If you can, lower the leg even more slowly.) Keep the knee straight. Relax. Repeat the entire legstretch sequence with the other leg.

Breathing. Breathe normally.

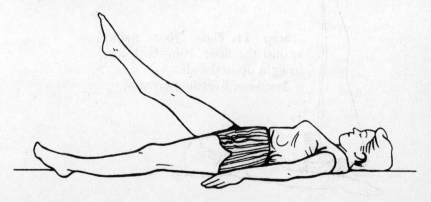

Step 8. Clasp both knees to your chest and hold for a count of eight.

Breathing. Inhale as you bring your knees to your chest.

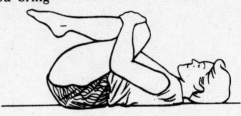

Step 9. Bring your head to your knees and hold for a count of eight.

Breathing. Exhale as you raise your head.

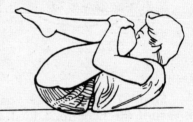

Step 10. Very slowly roll back down to the floor.

Breathing. Breathe normally.

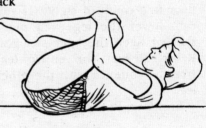

Step 11. Place your palms against the floor. Point both legs straight up in the air.

Breathing. Breathe normally.

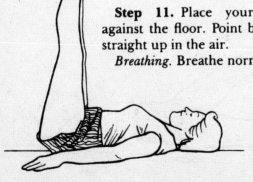

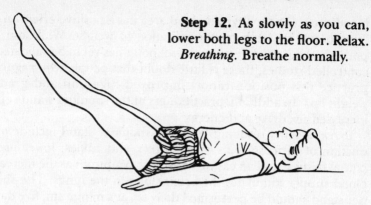

Step 12. As slowly as you can, lower both legs to the floor. Relax. *Breathing.* Breathe normally.

ADDITIONAL BENEFITS OF THE KNEES-TO-CHIN POSE

In addition to relieving flatulence and indigestion, the knees-to-chin pose helps to:

- Develop your ability to hold air in your lungs, which makes it an excellent adjunct to aerobics. It is also a good pose for those with asthma.
- Improve flexibility of the hip joints.
- Strengthen abdominal muscles.
- Strengthen leg muscles.
- Massage internal organs.

TWO KEY FULL-BODY STRETCHING POSES

THE SHOULDER STAND

This is perhaps the most important position in the entire array of stretching movements. According to experienced yogis who have mastered yoga techniques, the shoulder stand helps to delay the aging process. They believe it does this by stimulating your endocrine system and by increasing the supply of blood and oxygen to the brain, pineal gland, pituitary gland, and thyroid gland.

The shoulder stand is an excellent adjunct to your weight-control program because it also stimulates the thyroid gland, which regulates your metabolism. We believe that the increased blood supply to the thyroid gland area has a positive effect on the "set point" that leads to normalization of weight. While our hypothesis about the effects on the set point has yet to be validated in controlled studies, there is little doubt that people who regularly practice this position report improved digestion and gradual weight loss. In addition, practitioners of the shoulder stand report increased sex drive and energy.

Extra benefits resulting from the shoulder stand include a reduction of varicose veins, swollen feet, and ankles; fewer menopausal flashes; and an easing of asthma symptoms as the increased blood supply stimulates the bronchioles in the lungs. The shoulder stand should be performed daily or, at a minimum, five days a week. **Warning:** If you have any blood pressure problems, do *not* do this pose.

HOW TO DO THE SHOULDER STAND

The aim of the shoulder stand is to invert the body and thereby trap blood in the thyroid gland area. If you are stiff or overweight, you can prop yourself up against a wall. The object is to "get there" without hurting yourself, no matter how long it takes.

Step 1. Lie on your back with your palms flat on the floor. Stiffen your legs and use your abdominal muscles to raise your legs so they point at the ceiling.
Breathing. Breathe normally throughout this pose.

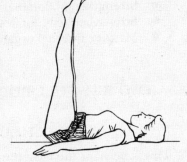

Step 2. Continue to bring your legs toward and over your head. Push down hard with your palms as you begin to raise your waist and hips off the floor.

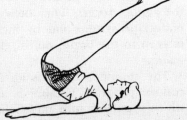

Step 3. When your hips are as far off the floor as you can get them, bring your hands up to your back to give yourself support.

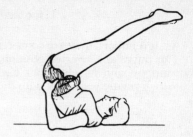

Step 4. Slowly straighten your back so that your weight is primarily on your shoulders. Your arms should form a triangle of support with your back. Your chin should be pressed into the hollow of your throat. Hold for a count of sixteen. Work up to a count of sixty-four. Advanced students hold for several minutes.

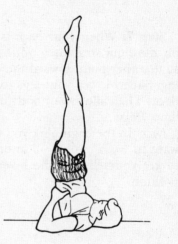

Step 5. Coming out of the shoulder stand properly is as important as getting into it. Lower your legs toward your head and roll a few vertebrae onto the floor so that your weight is supported by your upper back and arms.

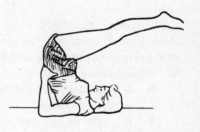

Step 6. When you feel balanced, place your palms flat against the floor and slowly roll down. Use your fingertips to steady yourself as you roll down.

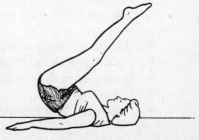

Visualization for Step 6

It is important not to come crashing down out of a shoulder stand (or out of any inverted position, for that matter). Use your arms for support and imagine your back as the roll-top desk. See yourself *slowly* rolling your back onto the floor one vertebra at a time.

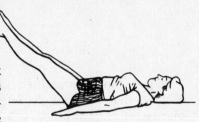

Step 7. When your back is flat on the floor, straighten your legs so that they point toward the ceiling. Slowly lower your legs to the floor. Then allow your body to go limp. Relax.

Note: In the beginning you may want to "walk" up a wall in order to get yourself into the inverted position.

THE COBRA

This pose helps keep your spine flexible and stimulates your abdominal organs, adrenal glands, and sex glands. In addition to increasing sexual energy and keeping the spine flexible, the cobra has the following benefits:

- It stimulates the pancreas, liver, and other organs of the digestive system.
- It alleviates constipation, indigestion, dysentery, flatulence, stomachaches, and other abdominal ailments. You may well find yourself "burping" as you finish this pose.
- It increases lung capacity and breath control.
- It strengthens heart and lungs.
- It stimulates the chest, shoulders, neck, and face.
- It firms the bust.
- It tightens back muscles and strengthens the back.

HOW TO DO THE COBRA

Step 1. Lie flat on your stomach with your head turned to one side. Put your hands at shoulder level with the fingers pointing toward your head. Relax, then put your forehead on the floor.

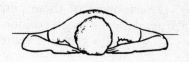

Step 2. Begin to roll your eyes up toward the ceiling. Inhale slowly and at the same time lift your head and upper body off the floor.

Breathing. Inhale as you raise off the floor.

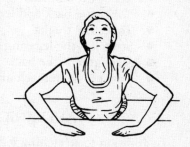

Visualization for Step 2

One of the tricks to this movement is to roll the eyes slowly up and back as you perform it. Visualize yourself looking up and back over the top of your head.

Step 3. Arch your head and upper back toward your heels. Hold for a count of eight. Work up to a count of sixteen.

Breathing. Hold your breath.

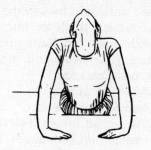

Step 4. Exhale as you slowly return to starting position. Allow your eyes to return to a normal position as you lower your upper body. Relax with cheek on floor.

Breathing. Exhale.

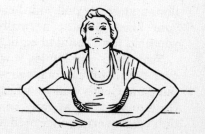

LEG STRETCHES AND PULLS

Practitioners of these positions report the following benefits from daily use. Each position

- Helps keep the spine flexible (helps especially after running)
- Helps correct constipation
- Tones the stomach
- Tones the back and legs
- Tones the thighs
- Stretches the legs and feet
- Strengthens the back
- Gets rid of stomach and thigh flab

ALTERNATE LEG PULLS

In addition to stretching leg muscles, alternate leg pulls stretch the Achilles tendons, and thus are an excellent routine for runners, swimmers, and cyclists.

HOW TO DO ALTERNATE LEG PULLS

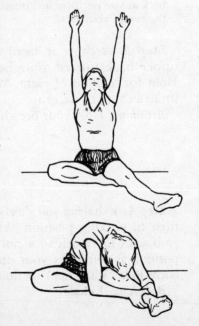

Step 1. Sit on the floor and place your right foot on the inside of your left thigh as close to the crotch as you can. Raise your arms above your head and inhale as you bend backward.

Breathing. Inhale.

Step 2. Twist toward your left leg and bend forward. Grab your left ankle with both hands. Exhale as you lower your elbows to the floor and gently pull your head to your knee. Breathe normally as you hold for a count of eight.

Note: Grab your left leg at whatever point you can manage without pain. Gently pull your head as close to your leg as you can, but don't be overly concerned with touching your knee in the beginning. It will come with time and practice.

Breathing. Exhale

Step 3. Slowly release your ankle and curl back up to a sitting position. Repeat with the other leg.

Breathing. Breathe normally.

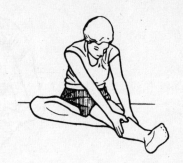

LEG STRETCHES

Leg stretches help keep the spine flexible. They tone the back, legs, and stomach, and reportedly help correct constipation.

HOW TO DO LEG STRETCHES

Step 1. Sit on the floor with your legs together. Inhale slowly as you raise your arms above your head and bend backward. The purpose of bending backward is to give the spine maximum stretch in preparation for the next step.

Breathing. Inhale.

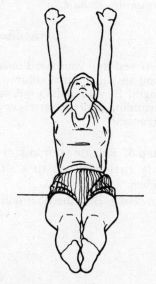

Visualization for Step 1

Imagine your spine being stretched gently to its maximum length, with lots of space between the vertebrae.

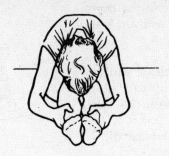

Step 2. Exhale as you bend forward and grab your ankles. Lower your elbows to the floor and slowly pull your head to your knees. Breathe normally while you hold for a count of eight.

Note: You may not be able to reach your ankles until you develop more flexibility. No matter. Grab your legs anywhere you can reach, even if it is only your knees. We guarantee that if you keep practicing this pose you will eventually be able to reach your ankles.

Breathing. Exhale.

Visualization for Step 2

As you pull your head toward your knees, imagine the rubber band in your spinal column stretching gently to its maximum length. In your mind's eye, see the spaces between the vertebrae expanding and the vertebrae themselves being pulled gently into alignment.

Step 3. Release your ankles and slowly curl back up to a sitting position.
Breathing. Breathe normally.

KNEELING POSITIONS

The classic kneeling positions are called the diamond and the child poses. Both are relatively easy to master. They are designed to strengthen your knees, ankles, and insteps. The diamond pose also helps to correct rheumatisim, stimulate the reproductive system, and to improve prolapsed uterus problems in women and enlarged prostate problems in men.

THE DIAMOND POSE

Step 1. Sit on your heels, with your back held straight. Place your hands on your knees. Close your eyes and concentrate on filling your body with energy.
Breathing. Breathe in and out slowly and rhythmically.

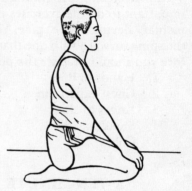

Note: The diamond pose can be adapted to reduce hemorrhoids and tone the vaginal muscles. When you are in the diamond pose inhale, exhale, and tighten the muscles of the anus (and, for women, the vagina), drawing them up into the body. Hold for a few seconds and relax. Repeat.

THE CHILD POSE

Step 1. Sit on your heels. Lean forward and put your forehead on the floor. Put your arms at your sides with the palms facing up.
Breathing. Breathe in and out slowly.

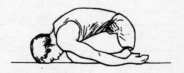

ADDITIONAL BENEFITS OF THE CHILD POSE

In addition to helping you relax and strengthening your knees, ankles, and insteps, the child pose has the following benefits:

- It relaxes the spine.
- It sends blood to the face and head.
- It tones the solar plexus.

A TWENTY-MINUTE DAILY STRETCHING PROGRAM

In a stretching program such as we have just described, it is important to do the exercises in an order that allows for complementary flexing of the spine. You want to follow a pose that flexes the spine forward with one that flexes the spine backward. Therefore you should practice the poses in the following order:

1. Hands to floor
2. Chest expansion
3. Knees to chin
4. Shoulder stand
5. Cobra
6. Alternate leg pulls
7. Leg stretches
8. Diamond pose
9. Child pose

A TEN-MINUTE DAILY PERSONAL STRETCHING PROGRAM

You will probably need to allow fifteen to twenty minutes to complete all nine poses. If you are pressed for time, remember that a little yoga is better than none. You can cut the time to ten minutes a day by doing the movements in Group A one day and those in Group B the next:

	Posture/ Movement	Group A	Group B
1.	Hands to floor	X	
2.	Chest expansion		X
3.	Knees to chin	X	
4.	Shoulder stand	X	X
5.	Cobra		X
6.	Alternate leg pulls	X	
7.	Leg stretches		X
8.	Diamond pose	X	
9.	Child pose		X

Chapter 22

Breathing the Right Way Will Give You a Natural High

You can live for months without food, for days without water, but you can live only a few minutes without oxygen. This chapter gives you an overview of the art and science of breathing for increased energy and health. The techniques described in this chapter will

- Increase your production of the high-energy molecule ATP
- Conserve your energy by helping you obtain oxygenated blood more efficiently
- Help you control stress
- Strengthen your immune system
- Improve your bowel functioning

THE FIVE BENEFITS OF LEARNING BREATH CONTROL

BENEFIT #1: YOU CAN MAKE MORE ENERGY MOLECULES

The energy that sustains life is generated when the fats and carbohydrates we eat combine with the oxygen we breathe. As we explained earlier, this energy is stored in a specialized set of molecules of a compound called adenosine triphosphate, or ATP for short, made with the help of certain other protein molecules or enzymes. Obviously, the more oxygen you have available to combine with your food intake, the more energy you produce. In other words, the more ATP you have in your body, the higher your energy level will be. That's where the power of breath control comes in.

Simply put, the greater your conscious control over your breathing, the more oxygen you can bring to your energy system. The breathing methods described in this chapter will increase the oxygen in your blood.

BENEFIT #2: INCREASED EFFICIENCY OF YOUR HEART-LUNG SYSTEM

There are two basic ways to breathe. Your body uses the same amount of oxygen whichever one you use. The main difference between the two methods lies in the amount of energy you save in processing your oxygen intake. One way to breathe is with your chest; the other is with your diaphragm.

Using your diaphragm is the most efficient and beneficial way to breathe. We call this "tummy" breathing. Children breathe this way naturally. Unfortunately, most of us acquire bad breathing habits (just as we acquire bad posture) as we grow up. We become chest breathers. According to Dr. Phil Nuernberger, writing in his book *Freedom from Stress*, you can cut the work load on your heart-lung system in half if you learn to be a tummy breather rather than a chest breather. You will be using only half as much of your energy reserves to take in the same amount of oxygen!

BENEFIT #3: YOU CAN IMPROVE CONTROL OF YOUR STRESS RESPONSE

Imagine walking alone down a dark street late at night. Suddenly you hear footsteps close behind you. Without your having to think about it, a complex interaction of physical changes takes place within your body. Your heart beats faster, your blood pressure rises, you breathe more quickly, your metabolism increases— all to speed more oxygen and nutrients to your cells. Your muscles tense, ready to serve as a kind of body armor and also to prepare you to spring from danger. Your blood platelets mobilize their clumping ability to help stop bleeding if you are wounded. All of these are part of your fight-or-flight response, the natural defense mechanism that gears up your body to deal with potential danger.

For many people a verbal fight with a spouse or a coworker produces the same physiological changes as the threat of physical attack. For others, just opening bills or receiving an upsetting phone call may bring about the same response. But the geared-up body has no place to run to, no target to strike, no physical outlet. Instead of helping, the storm of inner activity congeals into stress. Since chest breathing is under your control, when you regulate and slow down your breathing you can consciously break the stress response cycle as it is happening. And without tranquilizers!

BENEFIT #4: YOU CAN STRENGTHEN YOUR IMMUNE SYSTEM

Stress depresses your immune system. When your immune system is chronically depressed, you are more susceptible to illness. Fortunately, a slow and controlled pattern of breathing is one way to directly strengthen your immune system. When you are breathing slowly and rhythmically you increase alpha brain waves, which in turn induce a state of deep relaxation and increase the oxygenation of the blood—physical changes that help to build up your immune system.

BENEFIT #5: YOUR WASTE ELIMINATION SYSTEM WORKS BETTER

Diaphragmatic (tummy) breathing is a form of internal massage that, in effect, moves your internal organs up and down and increases the flow of blood to them. Tummy breathing also helps to stimulate the rhythmic, wavelike motion of the intestinal track (called peristalsis). This helps your body get rid of toxic wastes more efficiently.

SIX EASY STEPS TO DEEP DIAPHRAGMATIC BREATHING

Any time you need more energy or simply want to relax, follow these steps and enjoy:

Step 1. Fill your lungs.

Slowly breathe in. Draw the air into your abdomen and feel your stomach expand like a big balloon.

Step 2. Fill your chest.

In the same breath, continue to fill your lungs until your chest expands.

Step 3. Fill the top of your lungs.

Still as part of this continuous breath, raise your shoulders and fill the top of your lungs with air. Pull your shoulders up and back to make room for the air.

Step 4. Empty the top of your lungs.

Start exhaling by forcing the air from the upper portion of your lungs as you lower your shoulders. This empties the top third of your lungs.

Step 5. Empty your chest.

Next, push the air slowly out of the middle of your lungs by pulling in your chest.

Step 6. Empty your stomach.

Finally, push your stomach in to force all of the air out of your lungs. Relax. Now begin the cycle again.

YOUR NOSE KNOWS

Feeling depressed? Anxious? Want a way to handle depression or anxiety without drugs? Try alternate nostril breathing! Some recent research links certain emotional states with which side of your nose you usually use to exhale. For example, depressed people tend to breathe more out of the left nostril. Conversely, highly anxious people tend to breathe more out of the right nostril. To bring yourself into emotional balance, try using the technique of *alternate nostril breathing*. It has been used as a form of therapy for depression and anxiety.

HOW TO RELAX: ALTERNATE NOSTRIL BREATHING

Step 1: Right nostril breath.

Hold your left nostril closed with your index finger. Inhale through your right nostril. Exhale through your mouth. (*Optional:* Move your index finger to the other side of your nose and exhale through your left nostril.)

Step 2: Left nostril breath.

Hold your right nostril closed with your index finger. Draw in air through your left nostril. Exhale through your mouth. (*Op-*

tional: Move your index finger to the other side of your nose and exhale through your right nostril.)

Step 3: Repeat alternate nostril breathing until you feel relaxed.

QUICK ENERGY CHARGE #16

BREATH COUNTING

Steps 1–5: See the instructions preceding Quick Energy Charge #1 in chapter 4.

Step 6: Energy programming

Breathing slowly and deeply, see the oxygen entering every cell in your body. See your tiredness and tension melting into the grass, leaving you relaxed and alert. With each breath, breathe in increased energy and breathe out tiredness and stress. See the energy come into your body as pure white light.

Now that your deepest self is tuned in and harmonizing in this relaxed but alert state, begin to count your breathing cycles. As you breathe in, count to four. As you breathe out, count to eight. You should always take twice as long to breathe out as you do to breathe in. If "four" and "eight" are too much for you. Try "three" and "six". Remember to "tummy" breathe!

Continue the breath counting until you feel ready to go back to your everyday world. Then see yourself becoming more alert and more energetic because of your controlled breathing. In your mind's eye, see your face relaxed and without tension lines, see your eyes bright and alert, and see your mouth smiling.

Step 7: Reentry. See the instructions preceding Quick Energy Charge #1 in chapter 4.

Part V

ENERGY-BUILDING FOOD CHOICES

Chapter 23

Five-Star Recipes for the Seven-Day Program

Most of the recipes in this chapter were developed in cooperation with Chef Daniel Bumgardner. Chef Bumgardner has performed his culinary magic in numerous well-known gourmet restaurants from southern California to Rio de Janeiro to Florida. These include Sheffield's and Windows on the Green in Fort Lauderdale, Florida, and, most recently, the Champagne Room at LaCosta Hotel and Spa in Carlsbad, California. David and Joely did the meal planning and the computer-based nutritional analyses for the recipes and daily nutritional scorecards. The analyses were done with the help of Michael Jacobson's Nutrition Wizard™, a software program published by the Center for Science in the Public Interest (1986).

RECOMMENDED COLD CEREALS

Most of us have been conditioned to the notion that cereal with milk and fruit is a healthy breakfast. Actually, it may or may not be a healthy breakfast, depending on the quality of the ingredients you choose. Whole milk contains too much fat. The typical supermarket cereal is loaded with sugar and artificial ingredients. Although the largest selection of energy-building cold cereals is available in health food stores, this situation is beginning to change. As supermarkets get enough requests for healthy foods they are beginning to stock them. The cereals below meet the healthy, energy-building criteria of the Never Be Tired Again program:

HEALTH FOOD STORE CHOICES

Health Valley brand flakes:
- Stoned Wheat Flakes
- Oat Bran Flakes with almonds and dates
- Fiber 7 Flakes
- Golden Wheat Fruit Lites
- Golden Corn Fruit Lites
- Brown Rice Fruit Lites
- Amaranth Flakes

Health Valley brand granola-type:
- Sprouts 7 with Bananas & Hawaiian Fruit
- Wheat Germ & Fiber with Bananas & Tropical Fruit
- Sprouts 7 with Raisins
- Natural Sprouted Cereal with Amaranth

New Morning brand:
- Oatios
- Fruit-e-O's
- Crispy Brown Rice

Arrowhead Mills brand:
- Agrain and Agrain

Perky's brand:
- Apple & Cinnamon Crispy Brown Rice

Kashi Co. brand:
- Puffed Kashi

SUPERMARKET CHOICES

Nabisco brand
- Shredded Wheat

Quaker brand
- Puffed Wheat
- Puffed Rice

RECOMMENDED HOT CEREALS

Many healthy hot cereals are available in both health food stores and supermarkets. If you don't find a particular brand in your local supermarket, try a health food store:
- American Prairie Porridge Oats (our favorite)
- American Prairie Creamy Rye & Rice

- Lundberg's Creamy Brown Rice
- Nabisco Cream of Wheat (*not* instant)
- Nabisco Cream of Rice (*not* instant)
- Wheatena (hot)
- Quaker Oats
- Quick-Malt-O-Meal
- Albers Quick Grits
- Arrowhead Mills Rice & Shine
- McCann's Irish Oatmeal

RECOMMENDED SNACKS FOR CONSTANT ENERGY

Snacks are an important element in the Never Be Tired Again program. They help to keep your blood sugar on an even keel, constantly providing you with energy. Not only that, snacks will help prevent sugar and alcohol cravings as well as keep you from overeating at lunch and dinnertime.

Don't worry about calories. Remember, our motto is that you can eat all you want as long as you follow the five rules of the Never Be Tired Again nutrition program given in chapter 7. The point is, please eat the snacks recommended in your seven-day program. They are essential. Choose from this list:

GRAIN PRODUCTS

RICE CAKES

Choose any good, sodium-free brand. If you don't like them plain, use a teaspoon of one of the Never Be Tired Again approved jams as a topping. Our favorite rice cakes are made by the Lundberg family in California.

CRACKERS

The crackers listed below are low in fat and salt and have no additives or refined sugar:

Edward & Sons brand
- Zesty Parmesan Brown Rice Snaps (Dave's favorite)
- Onion Garlic Brown Rice Snaps
- Tamari Seaweed Brown Rice Snaps
- Buckwheat Brown Rice Snaps

Other Crackers
- Kavli

- Wasa Crispbread
- Ak-Mak
- Hol-Grain Whole Wheat, Lite Snack Thins

Pacific Rice Products brand
- Raisin 'N Spice Crispy Cakes
- Apple Cinnamon Crispy Cakes
- Chili'N Cheese Crispy Cakes
- Italian Spices Crispy Cakes

RECOMMENDED FRUIT AND FRUIT PRODUCTS

Fresh fruits not only supply you with vitamins, minerals, and fiber, they also help to curb "sugar cravings" at snack time. Some fruits have been shown to help lower cholesterol because of the pectin content. All fruits (except avocados and olives) are okay to eat. You can eat two or three pieces of fruit a day as a snack. Make sure that at least two come from this list:

- Apples
- Bananas
- Pears

JAMS

Most of the jams and jellies you are accustomed to are loaded with refined sugar. Jams or "conserves" made from pure fruit are delicious! The brands listed below contain no additives, sugar, or other ingredients. They are made from pure fruit:

- R. W. Knudsen
- Polaner All-Fruit
- Smucker's Simply Fruit brand—be careful that you don't accidentally buy their jams with refined sugar.
- Sorrell Ridge Fruit Only brand. Sorrell Ridge also makes a product that has honey in it. Make sure you buy the "fruit-only" variety.
- Westbrae Natural

RECOMMENDED BEVERAGES

- Water-process decaffeinated coffee. You can buy the beans and grind them at home or have them ground in the store. The brand names vary, but look for the "water-process" label. Drink your decaffeinated coffee black or with nonfat milk—no sugar! Try to avoid artificial sweeteners as well (see chapter 12).

- Decaffeinated tea with nonfat milk or lemon—no sugar.
- Carbonated waters (low-sodium, naturally carbonated preferred).
- Flavored carbonated waters. Make sure you read the label. You want the ones that are sugar-free, salt-free, and free of artificial ingredients.
- Herb teas (caffeine-free only).
- Spring water (not less than eight glasses per day).

THE SEVEN-DAY PROGRAM SHOPPING LIST

Grain products

Oatmeal
100% whole wheat flour
100% whole wheat pastry flour
Quinoa (See recipe #11. Available in most health food stores.)
Whole wheat spaghetti
Fettucine (DeBoles artichoke preferred)
Long grain brown rice
DeBoles artichoke lasagna
100% whole wheat bread
100% whole wheat rolls

Wine (optional)

Dry sherry
White table wine

Fruits, frozen, unsweetened

Strawberries
Raspberries
Blueberries
Peaches

Oils

Light olive oil

Sweeteners

Fruit concentrate (We prefer Mystic Lake Dairy,[3] but any unsweetened juice concentrate is okay.)
Unsweetened apple juice

Spices and herbs[1]

Bay leaf
Garlic powder
Chervil
Savory
Onion powder
Parsley
Finely ground black pepper
Chili powder
Cumin seed
Oregano
Cayenne
Coriander
Dry mustard
Red pepper
Tabasco
Basil
Tarragon
Thyme
Gourmet Sprinkle[2] or other herbal seasoning such as Mrs. Dash
Seafood Sprinkle[2] or other herbal seasoning such as Mrs. Dash

Dairy products

Skim milk
1% milk
Egg whites (from fresh eggs)
Low-fat cottage cheese
Nonfat yogurt
Feta cheese
Parmesan cheese, grated

Legumes[4]

Chickpeas (garbanzo beans)
Red kidney beans
Pinto beans
Split peas

Other cooking, baking ingredients

Baking powder (aluminum-free)
Broth (Vecon vegetable broth preferred. You can also use Pritikin's defatted chicken broth.)
Dijon mustard (regular or country)
Prepared mustard
Cornstarch
Apple cider vinegar
Red wine vinegar
Ginger root (fresh)
16-ounce can of tomatoes (no salt)
Bottled clam broth
Soy sauce or tamari—low-sodium

Fruits, fresh

Lemons
Oranges
Apples
Bananas
Pears

Vegetables for flavor

Onions
Scallions
Garlic

Vegetables for cooking and salads

White potatoes
Sweet potatoes or yams
Tomatoes
Bell peppers
Mushrooms
Celery
Carrots
Zucchini
Mung sprouts
Alfalfa sprouts
Lettuce, all (except iceberg)
Spinach
Chard
Radishes
Winter squash
Cucumbers

Commercial salad dressings[5]

Pritikin dressings

---

[1] In many of the recipes, fresh herbs are preferred.

[2] See chapter 12 for information on salt substitutes and Gourmet Sprinkle and Seafood Sprinkle. To order, write to: Potluck & Thyme, P.O. Box 1546, Salem, NH 03079-1546, or call 603-893-9965.

[3] See chapter 12 for information on fruit concentrates. Call 206-868-2029 for your nearest distributor.

[4] Home-cooked, from dry beans preferred. If you buy canned beans, make certain that they contain no added salt, preservatives, or artificial ingredients.

[5] If you want to try one of the commercial "lite brands," read the label carefully. Most contain preservatives, artificial flavors, and sodium.

The Recipes

HOT CEREAL WITH RAISINS
Recipe 1
Number of servings: 1

1 serving	hot cereal (See list of recommended cereals.)
2 Tbsp.	raisins
Dash	cinnamon
1 Tbsp.	oat bran
1 Tbsp.	fruit concentrate (Mystic Lake Dairy or apple concentrate*)

1. Cook cereal according to directions. Do *not* add salt. Add raisins and a dash of cinnamon to cereal as it cooks. Pour into bowl, add oat bran, and mix well. Top with fruit concentrate (or mix in 1 tablespoon of your favorite fruit-only jam).

*See shopping list at the beginning of this chapter.

NUTRITIONAL SCORECARD
Calories per serving: 296

NUTRIENT	Carbohydrate	Fat	Total Protein	Animal Protein	Sodium
PERCENT CALORIES	77%	10%	13%	0	
AMOUNT	57.1 G	3.2 G	9.8 G	0 G	9 mg.

COLD CEREAL WITH FRUIT
Recipe 2
Number of servings: 1

1 oz.	dry cereal (See list of recommended cereals.)
½ cup	nonfat milk
1	banana or ½ cup other fruit, such as strawberries or blueberries.
1 Tbsp.	oat bran

NUTRITIONAL SCORECARD
Calories per serving: 319

NUTRIENT	Carbohydrate	Fat	Total Protein	Animal Protein	Sodium
PERCENT CALORIES	78%	9%	13%	5%	
AMOUNT	64 G	3.2 G	11 G	4 G	72 mg.

EGG WHITE OMELETTE
Recipe 3

Number of servings: 1

3	egg whites
2	mushrooms, sliced (or to taste)
⅛–¼	onion, diced (or to taste)
¼	green pepper (or to taste)

1. Spray small nonstick skillet with cooking spray. Sauté onions, mushrooms, and peppers (or any combination you prefer) until tender. Add small amounts of water as needed to prevent sticking. You can make the vegetables in quantity and freeze individual portions in zip-top freezer bags. Once the vegetables are cooked, the omelette takes only a few minutes to make.

2. Separate three eggs, keeping the whites. Spray nonstick omelette pan with cooking spray. Pour egg whites into pan and cook over medium-high heat. When whites have solidified, remove from heat and place pan under broiler for 10 to 15 seconds to cook "inside" of omelette thoroughly. Add sautéed vegetables to pan. Fold the omelette in half and serve. It will be golden brown on the "outside" of the omelette. Garnish with salsa to make a Spanish Omelette if you like.

NUTRITIONAL SCORECARD
Calories per serving: 59

NUTRIENT	Carbohydrate	Fat	Total Protein	Animal Protein	Sodium
PERCENT CALORIES	23%	2%	75%	61%	
AMOUNT	57.1 G	3.2 G	9.6 G	9 G	9 mg.

OATMEAL PANCAKES
Recipe 4

Number of servings: 4
(makes 12–16 four-inch pancakes)

1 cup	uncooked oatmeal
1⅛ cups	skim milk (nonfat) or fruit juice
4	egg whites
½ cup	whole-wheat flour or oat flour
2 Tbsp.	fruit concentrate (Mystic Lake Dairy or apple concentrate*)
1 Tbsp.	aluminum-free baking powder

1. Soak oatmeal in milk for 5 minutes or so.
2. Stir in the egg whites, flour, fruit concentrate, and baking powder.
3. Heat nonstick griddle and spray with cooking spray. Bake pancakes on a hot griddle, turning when the top is bubbly and the edges are slightly dry. Respray griddle before pouring more batter.
4. Top pancakes with Fruit Topping (recipe #43) or unsweetened applesauce. Extra pancakes can be frozen.

*See shopping list at the beginning of this chapter.

NUTRITIONAL SCORECARD					
Calories per serving: 202					
NUTRIENT	Carbohydrate	Fat	Total Protein	Animal Protein	Sodium
PERCENT CALORIES	70%	9%	21%	10%	
AMOUNT	35.2 G	2.1 G	10.6 G	5.3 G	320 mg.

BLUEBERRY PANCAKES
Recipe 5

Number of servings: 4
(makes 12–16 four-inch pancakes)

1 cup	uncooked oatmeal
1⅛ cup	skim milk (nonfat) or fruit juice
4	egg whites
½ cup	whole-wheat flour or oat flour
2 Tbsp.	fruit concentrate (Mystic Lake Dairy or apple concentrate*)
1 Tbsp.	aluminum-free baking powder
½–1 cup	fresh or frozen blueberries, unsweetened

1. Soak oatmeal in milk for 5 minutes or so.
2. Stir in the egg whites, flour, fruit concentrate, and baking powder.
3. Add the blueberries. If you are using frozen fruit, first defrost and drain off excess liquid.
4. Heat nonstick griddle and spray with cooking spray. Bake pancakes on a hot griddle, turning when the top is bubbly and the edges are slightly dry. Respray griddle before pouring more batter. Top pancakes with Fruit Topping (recipe #43) or unsweetened applesauce. Extra pancakes can be frozen.

*See shopping list at the beginning of this chapter.

NUTRITIONAL SCORECARD					
Calories per serving: 236					
NUTRIENT	Carbohydrate	Fat	Total Protein	Animal Protein	Sodium
PERCENT CALORIES	73%	8%	19%	9%	
AMOUNT	42.6 G	2.1 G	11.1 G	5.25 G	126 mg.

BANANA RAISIN PANCAKES
Recipe 6

Number of servings: 4
(makes 12–16 four-inch pancakes)

1 cup	uncooked oatmeal
1⅛ cup	skim milk (nonfat) or fruit juice
4	egg whites
½ cup	whole-wheat flour or oat flour
2 Tbsp.	fruit concentrate (Mystic Lake Dairy or apple concentrate*)
1 Tbsp.	aluminum-free baking powder
¼ cup	raisins
½ to 1 cup	thinly sliced banana

1. Soak oatmeal in milk for 5 minutes or so.
2. Stir in the egg whites, flour, fruit concentrate, and baking powder.
3. Add banana and raisins to batter.
4. Heat nonstick griddle and spray with cooking spray. Bake pancakes on the hot griddle, turning when the top is bubbly and the edges are slightly dry. Respray griddle before pouring more batter.
5. Top pancakes with Fruit Topping (recipe #43) or unsweetened applesauce. Extra pancakes can be frozen.

*See shopping list at the beginning of this chapter.

NUTRITIONAL SCORECARD					
Calories per serving: 265					
NUTRIENT	Carbohydrate	Fat	Total Protein	Animal Protein	Sodium
PERCENT CALORIES	75%	8%	17%	8%	
AMOUNT	51.2 G	2.4 G	11.4 G	5.2 G	322 mg.

HEARTY VEGETABLE RAREBIT
Recipe 7

Number of servings: 6

This is so tasty that one of our "salt addict" friends volunteered that it didn't need a single grain of salt: "It's perfect the way it is." Extra servings make a wonderful addition to your selection of frozen meals and are delicious as a stuffing for baked potatoes.

Sauce:

1	medium acorn squash
1	thin-skinned white potato
1	sweet potato

Vegetables:

1	onion, chopped
1 cup	sliced broccoli
1 cup	sliced cauliflower
2	carrots, sliced
3	tomatoes, chopped, or 16 oz. canned tomatoes
3	garlic cloves, minced, or 3 tsp. prechopped
¼ tsp.	black pepper (or to taste)
1 tsp.	dried basil

Toast/topping:

6	slices whole-wheat toast (1 per person)
6 Tbsp.	grated Parmesan cheese (1 Tbsp. per person)

SAUCE:

1. Wash squash and potatoes well, then cut into chunks without peeling. (Acorn squash will cut more readily if you cook it briefly in the microwave or regular oven at moderate heat.) Steam squash and potatoes until soft (or use a pressure cooker).
2. Puree vegetables, skins and all. The skins add nice color and wonderful fiber to the sauce.

VEGETABLES:

3. Spray nonstick skillet with cooking spray. Sauté garlic and onions until onions are translucent. Add small amounts of water as needed to prevent sticking.
4. Add broccoli, cauliflower, carrots, tomatoes, and spices. Sauté.
5. Add sauce to vegetables and simmer until vegetables are cooked as desired.
6. Serve over whole-wheat toast. Sprinkle each serving with 1 tablespoon of grated Parmesan cheese.

NUTRITIONAL SCORECARD					
Calories per serving: 255					
NUTRIENT	Carbohydrate	Fat	Total Protein	Animal Protein	Sodium
PERCENT CALORIES	70%	14%	16%	4%	
AMOUNT	42 G	3.6 G	9.2 G	2 G	298 mg.

DOUBLE DECKER SANDWICH
Recipe 8

Number of servings: 1

2–4 Tbsp.	garbanzo spread (recipe #34)
4 slices	raw zucchini (or to taste)
2 slices	tomato (or to taste)
¼ cup	alfalfa sprouts (or to taste)
2 slices	whole-wheat toast

1. Spread a piece of toast with garbanzo spread.
2. Top with zucchini, tomato, and alfalfa sprouts. Add salsa if desired. Top with second piece of toast.

NUTRITIONAL SCORECARD
Calories per serving: 201

NUTRIENT	Carbohydrate	Fat	Total Protein	Animal Protein	Sodium
PERCENT CALORIES	67%	12%	21%	5%	
AMOUNT	34.6 G	2.8 G	10.7 G	2.3 G	443 mg.

TUNA BURGERS
Recipe 9

Number of servings: 4

1 6.5-oz can	tuna packed in water
½ cup	diced onions
½ cup	diced green pepper
2	celery stalks with leaves, diced
2 Tbsp.	uncooked oat bran
4	egg whites
½ cup	whole-wheat bread crumbs
½–1 tsp.	pepper (to taste)
1 tsp.	parsley
4	whole-wheat burger buns

1. Put the bread crumbs in a bowl. Mix in onion, green pepper, parsley, pepper, oat bran, and egg whites.
2. Drain water from canned tuna. Crumble tuna into bread mixture.
3. Form tuna mixture into 4 patties.
4. Heat nonstick skillet and spray with cooking spray. Cook the tuna burgers over moderate heat until golden brown on both sides.

5. Place each burger on a whole-wheat bun. Top with tomato slices, onion slices, and alfalfa sprouts. Serve with Hot Cha Cha Salsa or relish on the side.

| NUTRITIONAL SCORECARD
Calories per serving: 244 | | | | | |
NUTRIENT	Carbohydrate	Fat	Total Protein	Animal Protein	Sodium
PERCENT CALORIES	57%	13%	30%	12%	
AMOUNT	33.8 G	3.4 G	17.9 G	7.5 G	360 mg.

RIB-STICKING SPLIT PEA SOUP
Recipe 10

Number of servings: 8

Freeze extra servings in individual zip-top freezer bags for a quick meal when you don't have time to cook.

2 slices	nitrate-free bacon*
2 cups (1 lb.)	split green peas, well rinsed
6 cups	water
2	celery stalks with leaves, chopped
1	onion, chopped
2	large carrots, chopped
1	small purple turnip, chopped or 1 small sweet potato, chopped
1	clove garlic, minced, or 1 tsp. prechopped garlic
2	bay leaves
¼ tsp.	dried chervil
½ tsp.	dry savory
1 tsp.	dried basil

1. Brown bacon pieces and minced garlic together in soup pot. Stir occasionally to prevent sticking. Leave bacon drippings in the pot.
2. Add chopped vegetables to pot and cook until onion becomes translucent. Stir to prevent sticking.

*Bacon gets most of its calories from fat so, as a food, it is not part of the Never Be Tired Again program. It can, however, be used as a wonderful flavor enhancer for soups. Keep your bacon frozen so you won't be tempted to eat it. Instead of trying to peel off slices, simply cut across the end of the pound. Two thin cuts will give you about two pieces of bacon already cut into pieces.

3. Add water and rinsed split peas. Bring to a boil, then reduce heat.
4. Add bay leaves, chervil, savory, and basil. Simmer for about 1½ hours or until split peas are tender.
5. Use a potato masher to reduce vegetables to very small bits right in the cooking pot. If you prefer your soup to have a smoother consistency, puree small amounts of the soup in a blender or food processor until all of the vegetables have been pureed.
6. If soup becomes too thick as it cools, add more water. Unused soup can easily be frozen in individual servings in zip-top freezer bags or Seal-A-Meal bags.

NUTRITIONAL SCORECARD
Calories per serving: 246

NUTRIENT	Carbohydrate	Fat	Total Protein	Animal Protein	Sodium
PERCENT CALORIES	63%	14%	23%	1%	
AMOUNT	39.3 G	3.9 G	14.7 G	.5 G	66 mg.

QUINOA AND TOMATO SOUP*
Recipe 11 *Number of servings: 6*

Quinoa (pronounced *keen*-wa) is an exciting "new" grain from the Andean Mountain regions of South America and was one of the staple foods of the Incas. It contains more protein than any other grain and has an amino acid balance close to the ideal. It cooks very quickly (15 minutes) and can be used for almost any grain in almost any recipe. If you can't find it in your local health food store or supermarket, call 1-800-237-2304 for the name of your nearest distributor. You can substitute brown rice for the quinoa if you prefer.

Surprise your family with a delicious homemade soup that takes only a short time to make. It freezes very well so if you have any left, package it in individual servings and keep it for those hectic days when you don't have time to cook.

*Adapted with permission from the Quinoa Corporation, Boulder, Colorado

1	garlic clove, minced, or 1 tsp. prechopped garlic
1 tsp.	chopped fresh cilantro or parsley
1	onion, diced
½	green pepper, chopped
2	celery stalks, chopped
1	tomato, chopped
½ cup	uncooked quinoa or brown rice
6 cups	Vecon vegetable broth or defatted chicken broth (Or look for Pritikin's defatted chicken broth in your food store.)
1	scallion, sliced
2 Tbsp.	grated Parmesan cheese

1. Spray pot with cooking spray. Add garlic, onion, pepper, and celery. Stir to prevent sticking.
2. Add tomatoes and broth. Bring to a boil.
3. Rinse quinoa. Its natural coating can be somewhat bitter-tasting. The bitterness can be removed by simply rinsing well before cooking.
4. Add quinoa to pot and return to a boil. Reduce heat, cover and simmer for 30 minutes. Add cilantro and continue to simmer for an additional 15 minutes.
5. Garnish each bowl with scallion slices and 1 teaspoon grated cheese.

NUTRITIONAL SCORECARD
Calories per serving: 102

NUTRIENT	Carbohydrate	Fat	Total Protein	Animal Protein	Sodium
PERCENT CALORIES	65%	17%	18%	3%	
AMOUNT	16.5 G	1.9 G	4.6 G	.67 G	294 mg.

SPAGHETTI WITH SAUCE AND CHEESE
Recipe 12

Number of servings: 1

2 oz.	uncooked spaghetti (Use DeBoles Artichoke Pasta, whole-wheat pasta, or corn pasta.)
4 oz.	spaghetti sauce*
2 Tbsp.	Parmesan cheese, grated

1. When you boil pasta, do not add oil or salt to the water.
2. Serve with a generous salad and one of the approved dressings for a delicious and filling meal.

*Read the label on your favorite spaghetti sauce. You can use a sauce with up to 25 percent fat because it is balanced by the pasta. The analysis that follows is based on a sauce with 15 percent fat.

NUTRITIONAL SCORECARD					
Calories per serving: 310					
NUTRIENT	Carbohydrate	Fat	Total Protein	Animal Protein	Sodium
PERCENT CALORIES	67%	15%	18%	5%	
AMOUNT	49 G	5 G	13 G	4 G	216 mg.

QUICK AND TASTY FAJITAS
Recipe 13   *Number of servings:* 1

1	small garlic clove or ½ tsp. chopped garlic
½	small zucchini, cut into long strips
1	scallion, chopped (Use whole scallion.)
¼	tomato, chopped
1 oz.	chickpeas, mashed
2	mushrooms, sliced
1 Tbsp.	salsa (mild, medium, or hot to taste)
1	whole-wheat tortilla

1. Spray nonstick skillet with vegetable spray. Brown garlic lightly. Add vegetables and salsa. Sauté until zucchini is slightly crunchy.
2. Heat tortilla in nonstick skillet or microwave oven. When cooked, spoon onto tortilla, making a line down the center with the vegetables. Roll tortilla and enjoy.

NUTRITIONAL SCORECARD
Calories per serving: 164

NUTRIENT	Carbohydrate	Fat	Total Protein	Animal Protein	Sodium
PERCENT CALORIES	71%	13%	16%	0%	
AMOUNT	31.2 G	2.5 G	6.8 G	0 G	5 mg.

CHICKEN AND FETTUCINE
Recipe 14   *Number of servings:* 4

8 oz.	fettucine*
6 oz.	deboned, skinned chicken breast
4 cups	raw mushrooms
1	garlic clove, minced, or 1 tsp. prechopped garlic
¼ cup	pale dry sherry
¼ cup	Vecon vegetable broth or defatted chicken broth
½ cup	plain nonfat yogurt
½ cup	low-fat cottage cheese
2 Tbsp.	country Dijon mustard
1 tsp.	cornstarch, mixed with a little water
4	sprigs parsely

1. Slice chicken into thin strips.
2. Heat water for fettucine.
3. Spray nonstick skillet with cooking spray. Sauté minced garlic. Add sherry, broth, mushrooms, and sliced chicken to skillet. Cook on medium heat until chicken turns white.
4. Cook fettucine.
5. While chicken is cooking combine the nonfat yogurt, low-fat cottage cheese, and Dijon mustard in blender and puree until smooth.
6. Add cornstarch to chicken skillet and bring to a boil. Cook until thickened, then turn down heat.
7. Add yogurt, cottage cheese, and mustard mixture to skillet. Heat thoroughly.
8. Add fettucine to skillet and toss. Transfer to serving platter. Use kitchen scissors to cut parsley into flakes to top fettucine. Garnish with more parsley sprigs.

*Deboles Jerusalem artichoke fettucine with spinach makes a very healthy and colorful dish.

NUTRITIONAL SCORECARD					
Calories per serving: 447					
NUTRIENT	Carbohydrate	Fat	Total Protein	Animal Protein	Sodium
PERCENT CALORIES	47%	11%	38%	26%	
AMOUNT	51.8 G	5.1 G	42 G	29.2 G	364 mg.

SWEET AND SOUR CHICKEN WITH RICE
Recipe 15   *Number of servings:* 4

Meat:

2   deboned, skinless chicken breasts, cut into thin slices

Vegetables:

2   celery stalks, sliced on diagonal
2   carrots, sliced on diagonal
1   onion, chopped
½   bell pepper, sliced
1   tart green apple (e.g., Granny Smith) cut into chunks (with skin)
2   garlic cloves, minced

Sauce:

8 oz.   canned pineapple slices, packed in own juice
½ cup   papaya juice
½ cup   vinegar
2 Tbsp.   fruit concentrate (Mystic Lake Dairy or apple concentrate*)
2 Tbsp.   cornstarch, mixed with 3 Tbsp. water
½ tsp.   black pepper
1 cup   green seedless grapes
1 Tbsp.   prepared mustard

1. Spray nonstick skillet with cooking spray. Sauté chicken and onions over medium heat until chicken turns white and onions are tender. Add celery, carrots, onion, apple, and garlic to pan.
2. While chicken and vegetables are cooking, prepare sauce in another pan. Combine juice from canned pineapple, papaya juice, vinegar, mustard, pepper, and fruit concentrate. Bring to a boil.
3. Add cornstarch mixture to sauce, stirring constantly until thickened. Cut pineapple into chunks, then add pineapple chunks and grapes to sauce. Return to boil. When sauce is thickened, add sauce to chicken and vegetables.
4. Serve over cooked brown rice (recipe #27) or noodles.

*See shopping list in the beginning of this chapter.

NUTRITIONAL SCORECARD					
Calories per serving: 473					
NUTRIENT	Carbohydrate	Fat	Total Protein	Animal Protein	Sodium
PERCENT CALORIES	67%	6%	27%	25%	
AMOUNT	68 G	3.1 G	32.4 G	29.2 G	165 mg.

BEEF WITH BROCCOLI STIR-FRY
Recipe 16

Number of servings: 6

This recipe is an entire meal in itself. Don't be fooled by the long directions. It will be on the table in less than 30 minutes if the rice is cooked in advance. Because the recipe cooks so quickly, it's best to prepare all ingredients in advance.

Meat:

¾ lb.	flank steak, thinly sliced

Vegetables:

1	garlic clove, minced, or 1 tsp. prechopped garlic
2 slices	ginger root, minced, or 1 tsp. prechopped ginger
2 cups	chopped broccoli
1 cup	sliced mushrooms
2 cups	Mung bean sprouts (thick white sprouts)
1 cup	chopped onions
½ cup	canned water chestnuts or bamboo shoots
1	green or red pepper, sliced

Sauce:

1 cup	Vecon vegetable broth or defatted chicken broth
1 Tbsp.	soy sauce
1 Tbsp.	pale dry sherry wine
2 tsp.	sesame oil
¼ tsp.	black pepper (or to taste)
2 tsp.	cornstarch, mixed with 2 Tbsp. water

Rice:

2 cups	cooked brown rice or noodles

1. Cook brown rice if you don't have some frozen (see recipe #27).
2. Cut broccoli into bite-size pieces. Cut tough outer skin from stem. Slice stem into thin pieces. Instead of cutting straight down through stem, angle your knife and cut on the diagonal. This will give you a larger cooking surface on each piece and help to cook it more quickly.
3. Slice the flank steak on a slant into very thin slices.
4. Prepare the onion, pepper, mushrooms, garlic, and ginger.
5. Steam the broccoli until slightly crunchy.

6. While the broccoli is steaming, spray a large nonstick skillet (or wok) with cooking spray. Add chopped garlic and ginger, sliced onion, and sliced pepper. Stir frequently, adding small amounts of water as needed to prevent sticking. Cook until onions and peppers are tender.
7. Add sliced mushrooms, water chestnuts, and bean sprouts to vegetables. Turn down heat.
8. Heat a second skillet. Spray with cooking spray and add steak. Stir-fry until meat is cooked. It will take only a few minutes.
9. Combine ingredients for sauce. Add to vegetables and bring to boil so that it thickens.
10. Add steak to vegetable mixture. Toss well to coat. Serve over rice.

NUTRITIONAL SCORECARD					
Calories per serving: 231					
NUTRIENT	Carbohydrate	Fat	Total Protein	Animal Protein	Sodium
PERCENT CALORIES	49%	20%	30%	21%	
AMOUNT	28 G	5.5 G	18.1 G	12.3 G	266 mg.

*Alcohol contributes 1 percent of the calories.

VEGETABLE LASAGNA
Recipe 17

Number of servings: 8

This is not a difficult dish to prepare, but you can simplify the preparation even more by using your favorite prepared sauce. Just make sure it is no more than 25 percent fat according to the label. (See chapter 8 for directions on reading labels.) The chef suggests that the flavor in this dish definitely improves over time, so consider making this the night before.

Sauce:

3	garlic cloves, minced, or 3 tsp. prechopped
½	green pepper, minced
¼	onion, minced
28-oz. can	tomato puree
1 cup	burgundy or other dry red wine
1 Tbsp.	fruit concentrate (Mystic Lake Dairy; optional)
¼ tsp.	black pepper

Vegetables:

½ head	small cauliflower, sliced
1½ cups	sliced broccoli, well packed
1 cup	sliced zucchini
1 cup	sliced mushrooms

Filling:

1½ cups	low-fat (2%) cottage cheese
½ cup	chickpeas (garbanzo beans)—optional
2	garlic cloves, minced, or 1 tsp. prechopped

Lasagna noodles:

1 10-oz. pkg.	DeBoles Jerusalem artichoke lasagna noodles

Topping:

¼ cup	Parmesan cheese, grated

LASAGNA NOODLES:

1. Boil noodles until tender. Do not add any oil or salt to the cooking water. Drain and set aside.

SAUCE:

2. Add all ingredients for sauce to pan. Let simmer while you prepare filling. Or use your favorite prepared sauce.

FILLING:

3. Puree chickpeas in blender. Add cottage cheese and minced garlic and puree again.

PREPARATION:

4. Pour a little sauce to cover the bottom of lasagna pan. Add a layer of noodles, one-third of the vegetables, one-third of the filling, and some sauce. Continue making layers. End with noodles topped with sauce.

5. Bake covered at 350° for 30 minutes. Turn oven off. Sprinkle top with ¼ cup grated Parmesan cheese and let stand for 30 minutes in the oven.

6. If you cook this the night before, remove the lasagna from the oven after the initial 30-minute cooking period. Sprinkle with cheese and replace cover. When you want to serve, reheat covered at 300° for 30 minutes.

NUTRITIONAL SCORECARD Calories per serving: 297					
NUTRIENT	Carbohydrate	Fat	Total Protein	Animal Protein	Sodium
PERCENT CALORIES	64%	9%	21%	9%	
AMOUNT	47.8 G	2.8 G	15.9 G	6.8 G	256 mg.

POTATO PANCAKES
Recipe 18   *Number of servings:* 4; makes 8 pancakes

3	thin-skinned potatoes, with skin
1 cup	raw onions
3 cloves	garlic
1 tsp.	black pepper
3 Tbsp.	whole-wheat flour
2 oz.	uncooked oat bran
1 Tbsp.	chopped parsley
3	green onions, chopped (Use entire onion.)
2	egg whites

1. Grate together potatoes, onions, and garlic.
2. Mix green onions, pepper, parsley, oat bran, flour, and egg whites with potato onion mixture.
3. Spray nonstick griddle with cooking spray. Form batter into patties and grill until golden brown on each side.
4. Finish by putting pancakes in preheated 350° oven for 5 minutes to crisp.
5. Serve with applesauce or Healthy Sour Cream (recipe #37). In the nutritional analysis for this recipe the first number under a given category is for two pancakes with applesauce and the second number is for pancakes with Healthy Sour Cream.

NUTRITIONAL SCORECARD
Calories per serving: 249–284

NUTRIENT	Carbohydrate	Fat	Total Protein	Animal Protein	Sodium
PERCENT CALORIES	78–84%	3–5%	13–17%	3–6%	
AMOUNT	53.3–55.4 G	8–1.6 G	8–12.4 G	1.5–4.3 G	42–113 mg.

ZUCCHINI BEAN CASSEROLE
Recipe 19

Number of servings: 4

2 cups	grated zucchini
1 cup	grated onion
3	tomatoes (2 chopped, 1 sliced)
2–4	garlic cloves, minced
2 sprigs	fresh cilantro or ½ tsp. dried cilantro
3 cups	cooked kidney beans
3 oz.	salsa (We like Hot Cha Cha brand. Use mild, medium, or hot to suit your taste.)
½ cup	grated cheddar cheese
4	whole-wheat tortillas

1. Mix grated zucchini and onion together with minced garlic and chopped tomatoes.
2. Puree 2 cups of beans together with the salsa and cilantro.
3. Spray baking dish with cooking spray. Spread bottom of the dish with a little of the pureed bean mixture.
4. Break two of the tortillas into pieces and spread to cover bottom of dish.
5. Mix remaining whole beans into pureed bean mixture. Pour half of the mixed beans in dish. Add half the zucchini-onion-tomato mixture. Add half of the grated cheese.
6. Break the remaining two tortillas into pieces and spread to cover mixture in baking dish. Pour remaining bean mixture into dish. Add remaining zucchini-onion-tomato mixture. Top with remaining cheese. Arrange sliced tomato in pinwheel shape on top of the cheese as a garnish.
7. Cover and bake at 400° for 30 minutes. Remove from oven and let stand for 15 minutes.

NUTRITIONAL SCORECARD					
Calories per serving: 355					
NUTRIENT	Carbohydrate	Fat	Total Protein	Animal Protein	Sodium
PERCENT CALORIES	62%	17%	21%	16%	
AMOUNT	56 G	6.7 G	19.4 G	14 G	826 mg.

SAN DIEGO CHILI
Recipe 20

This recipe makes a very spicy chili if you use the maximum amount of the spices indicated. If you love chili but would prefer not to have a hot taste, use the smaller amount indicated for each spice.

Number of servings: 8–12

3 cups	cooked red kidney beans*
28-oz. can	tomatoes (no salt)
2 cups	chopped celery
2 cups	chopped onion
1	green pepper, chopped
2	carrots, chopped
2	whole tomatoes, chopped
3–6	garlic cloves, minced
1 tsp.–1 Tbsp.	chili powder
½–1 tsp.	dry mustard
¼–½ tsp.	crushed red pepper
½–1 tsp.	Tabasco
1 tsp.	black pepper
1 tsp.	thyme
2	bay leaves
¼ cup	chopped fresh parsley or 3 Tbsp. dried parsley
1 Tbsp.	basil
1 Tbsp.	grated cheese

1. Put all ingredients in a pot. Bring to a boil. Reduce heat, cover, and simmer approximately 45 minutes.
2. Cut a slit into a baked potato and stuff with the chili. Sprinkle with 1 tablespoon grated cheese.
3. Freeze leftover chili in individual servings. Reheat and serve over rice or noodles for a quick meal.

*If you buy canned beans, try to buy the no-salt kind. If you can't find a no-salt version, rinse beans thoroughly. Or cook your own.

NUTRITIONAL SCORECARD
Calories per serving: 295*

NUTRIENT	Carbohydrate	Fat	Total Protein	Animal Protein	Sodium
PERCENT CALORIES	86%	2%	12%	3%	
AMOUNT	65.5 G	.7 G	9.1 G	2 G	224 mg.

*Total calories are 350 for a serving stuffed into a baked potato with skin and 420 when served over ½ cup of brown rice.

POACHED SALMON IN WINE WITH TOMATO CAPER SAUCE
Recipe 21 *Number of servings:* 4

A very elegant dish that takes only fifteen minutes to prepare and cook.

Fish:

1 lb.	pink salmon steak
1 cup	white wine

Sauce:

1 16-oz. can	crushed tomatoes with no salt
3	garlic cloves, minced, or 1 Tbsp. prechopped garlic
2 Tbsp.	fresh tarragon or 2 tsp. dried
½ tsp.	black pepper
1 Tbsp.	capers
2 Tbsp.	fruit concentrate (Mystic Lake Dairy or apple concentrate)
2 Tbsp.	cornstarch, mixed with 3 Tbsp. water

FISH:
1. Remove skin from salmon by grasping fish firmly at smallest end. Slide a very sharp knife between fish and skin. Angle knife towards skin and slide towards wide end. As an alternative method of skinning the fish, you can wait until fish is cooked. Skin will peel off easily.
2. Put fish and wine in large skillet on top of stove. Cook on high for 4 to 6 minutes or until fish is firm and flakes separate easily. Set salmon aside on a serving platter. Save the cooking liquid.

SAUCE:
1. While salmon is cooking, combine crushed tomatoes, garlic, tarragon, pepper, capers, and fruit concentrate in a saucepan. Bring to a boil. Add liquid from fish as soon as fish is cooked.
2. Add cornstarch to sauce, stirring constantly. Cook until thickened.
3. Cut salmon into four pieces. Pour sauce over fish. Top with sprig of fresh tarragon.

NUTRITIONAL SCORECARD					
Calories per serving: 250					
NUTRIENT	Carbohydrate	Fat	Total Protein	Animal Protein	Sodium
PERCENT CALORIES	28%	17%	39%	36%	
AMOUNT	16.9 G	4.8 G	24.3 G	22.7 G	290 mg.

DELICIOUS FISH STEW
Recipe 22

Number of servings: 4

2 slices	nitrate-free bacon, diced
1	garlic clove, minced, or 1 tsp. preminced garlic
1 cup	chopped onions
2	carrots, chopped
2	medium potatoes, diced, (about 2 cups)
1 cup	chopped celery (2 stalks)
3 cups	bottled clam broth (or more, to taste)
½ tsp.	black pepper
¼ tsp.	thyme
1 tsp.	Seafood Sprinkle* or other herbal salt substitute
1 tsp.	basil
8 oz.	cod, cut into pieces
4 sprigs	fresh parsley or 2 tsp. dried parsley

1. Brown bacon. Leave bacon drippings in pan.
2. Brown garlic in bacon drippings.
3. Add chopped onions, potatoes, carrots, and celery to bacon. Sauté.
4. Add clam juice, pepper, thyme, Seafood Sprinkle, garlic, and basil. (Adjust seasonings to taste.)
5. Simmer until vegetables are tender.
6. Add fish and cook 5 to 8 minutes or until fish turns milky white and flakes easily.
7. Pour into soup bowls. Bunch parsley and use kitchen scissors to cut parsley into tiny flakes to top stew (or sprinkle dried parsley).

*See shopping list in the beginning of this chapter.

NUTRITIONAL SCORECARD					
Calories per serving: 204					
NUTRIENT	Carbohydrate	Fat	Total Protein	Animal Protein	Sodium
PERCENT CALORIES	48%	11%	41%	26%	
AMOUNT	24.5 G	2.4 G	20.5 G	13.64 G	131 mg.

POACHED FISH WITH SAUCE
Recipe 23   *Number of servings:* 4

1 lb.	halibut or other white fish
¼ cup	white wine (to cover bottom of pan)
1	garlic clove, minced, or 1 tsp. prechopped garlic
1 recipe	Lemony Wine and Tarragon Sauce (See recipe #42.)

1. Put fish and wine in skillet. Spread minced garlic over fish. Sauté over high heat until fish turns white and flakes easily (4 to 5 minutes depending on thickness of fish). Or put fish, wine, and garlic in covered oven-proof dish. Bake at 425° for 10 to 12 minutes.
2. Remove fish from skillet or dish. Arrange on platter and dress with lemony wine and tarragon sauce (or use other sauce of your choice). Garnish with parsley.

NUTRITIONAL SCORECARD
Calories per serving: 156

NUTRIENT	Carbohydrate	Fat	Total Protein	Animal Protein	Sodium
PERCENT CALORIES	7%	13%	78%	75%	
AMOUNT	2.5 G	2.2 G	29.6 G	29.2 G	80 mg.

FISH AND CHIPS
Recipe 24

Number of servings: 4

Chips:

3	potatoes, washed well
2	egg whites

Fish:

1 lb.	fresh Atlantic cod or flounder
3 slices	whole-wheat bread
¼ cup	whole-wheat flour
2	egg whites
2 Tbsp.	Seafood Sprinkle* or other herbal seasoning
¼ tsp.	black pepper

CHIPS:

1. Cut potatoes (with skin) into steak-fry size. Dip into egg whites.
2. Spray nonstick baking sheet with cooking spray. Lay potatoes on sheet and spray top of potatoes lightly with cooking spray.
3. Bake at 350° for 40 minutes, turning halfway through cooking time. Check to see that potatoes are crispy on the outside and thoroughly cooked inside.
4. Serve with rice vinegar for an English flavor or with a sugar-free ketchup such as Westbrae Natural's "Un-Ketchup."

FISH:

1. Put whole-wheat bread in blender and make into crumbs. Add pepper and Seafood Sprinkle to egg whites.
2. Cut fish into six to eight pieces. Roll fish lightly in whole-wheat flour, dip in seasoned egg white, and coat with bread crumbs. Press crumbs into fish firmly.
3. Spray nonstick cookie sheet with cooking spray. Arrange fish and bake at 350° for 30 minutes or until crisp.

*See shopping list in the beginning of this chapter.

NUTRITIONAL SCORECARD					
Calories per serving: 375					
NUTRIENT	Carbohydrate	Fat	Total Protein	Animal Protein	Sodium
PERCENT CALORIES	57%	5%	38%	29%	
AMOUNT	53.4 G	2.1 G	35.3 G	28.3 G	290 mg.

SCALLOPS WITH ARTICHOKE SAUCE AND RICE
Recipe 25 *Number of servings* 4

1 pkg.	frozen artichoke hearts, cooked and drained
2	tomatoes, chopped
3	garlic cloves, minced, or 3 tsp. prechopped
2 Tbsp.	nonfat yogurt
½ cup	onions, chopped
⅓ cup	cooking sherry
¼ tsp.	black pepper
1 lb.	scallops
1 slice	whole-wheat bread, made into crumbs in blender
2 cups	cooked brown rice (See recipe #27.)

1. Combine cooked artichoke hearts, halve the chopped tomato, and the yogurt in blender and lightly puree.
2. Spray nonstick skillet with cooking spray. Sauté garlic and onion, adding small amounts of water to prevent sticking.
3. Add pureed mixture, remaining chopped tomato, sherry, and pepper to skillet. Mix thoroughly.
4. Add scallops to skillet and mix thoroughly.
5. Pour scallops and sauce into baking dish. Top with bread crumbs and bake at 350° for 15 minutes. If necessary, turn on high broil for one minute at the end to brown bread crumbs.
6. Serve over rice.

NUTRITIONAL SCORECARD					
Calories per serving: 306					
NUTRIENT	Carbohydrate	Fat	Total Protein	Animal Protein	Sodium
PERCENT CALORIES	59%	3%	31%	23%	
AMOUNT	44.4 G	1.1 G	23.5 G	17.8 G	377 mg.

*Seven percent of the calories in this recipe come from the alcohol in the sherry.

SPINACH WITH TOMATOES AND FETA CHEESE
Recipe 26   *Number of Servings:* 4

1 bunch	fresh spinach or 1 10-oz. bag of frozen leaf spinach
3 cloves	garlic, minced, or 3 tsp. prechopped garlic
1 oz.	feta cheese (domestic has less salt than imported)
2	tomatoes

1. Cut each tomato into eight pieces.
2. Spray nonstick skillet with cooking spray. Sauté garlic.
3. Add spinach and tomato wedges. Because of the natural juices in the spinach and tomatoes, no oil or water is required.
4. Crumble feta cheese and add halfway through cooking.

NUTRITIONAL SCORECARD					
Calories per serving: 76					
NUTRIENT	Carbohydrate	Fat	Total Protein	Animal Protein	Sodium
PERCENT CALORIES	55%	19%	26%	4%	
AMOUNT	11.3 G	1.8 G	5.2 G	.17 G	171 mg.

BROWN RICE
Recipe 27   *Number of servings:* 4

1 cup	brown rice (We like long-grain brown rice.)
2 cups	water or vegetable or defatted chicken broth
	Herbal seasonings, to taste (Avoid seasoning salts.)

1. Add rice and seasonings of choice to cold water. Bring to a boil and boil for one minute. Cover and reduce heat to simmer. Cook for 35 minutes or until water is completely absorbed and rice is tender. Brown rice is a little chewier and more flavorful than white rice.

NUTRITIONAL SCORECARD					
Calories per serving: 111					
NUTRIENT	Carbohydrate	Fat	Total Protein	Animal Protein	Sodium
PERCENT CALORIES	87%	5%	8%	0%	
AMOUNT	23.9 G	.6 G	2.3 G	0 G	17 mg.

SWEET AND TANGY CARROTS
Recipe 28   *Number of servings:* 4

4	raws carrots, cut diagonally into ¼-inch slices
2 Tbsp.	Dijon mustard
2 Tbsp.	fruit concentrate (Mystic Lake Dairy* or apple concentrate)
2 sprigs	fresh parsley, chopped

1. Steam carrots 5 to 10 minutes, until crunchy. Drain well.
2. Stir in mustard and fruit concentrate; stir over medium heat 1 to 2 minutes, until carrots are glazed.
3. Sprinkle with parsley.

*See shopping list in the beginning of this chapter.

NUTRITIONAL SCORECARD					
Calories per serving: 59					
NUTRIENT	Carbohydrate	Fat	Total Protein	Animal Protein	Sodium
PERCENT CALORIES	81%	9%	10%	0%	
AMOUNT	12.4 G	.6 G	1.5 G	0 G	123 mg.

DOMINO POTATOES
Recipe 29

Number of servings: 4

2	white-skinned potatoes
¼ cup	Vecon vegetable broth or defatted chicken broth
1 tsp.	rosemary
⅛ tsp.	black pepper
½ tsp.	Gourmet Sprinkle* or other herbal seasoning
2 Tbsp.	whole-wheat bread crumbs

1. Wash potatoes thoroughly. Do not peel. Cut in half lengthwise. Cut each half into thin (⅛-inch) half-moon slices. Keep slices together so potato maintains its shape.
2. Arrange potatoes in rows (for a square baking dish) or in circles (for a round baking dish). Stagger pieces like fallen dominoes.
3. Sprinkle with herbs.
4. Pour broth down the side of the baking dish.
5. Bake, covered, at 350° for 25 minutes or until done.
6. Sprinkle with bread crumbs. Brown under high broil for 1 minute.

*See shopping list in the beginning of this chapter.

NUTRITIONAL SCORECARD					
Calories per serving: 74					
NUTRIENT	Carbohydrate	Fat	Total Protein	Animal Protein	Sodium
PERCENT CALORIES	85%	3%	12%	0%	
AMOUNT	15.8 G	.2 G	2.1 G	0 G	84 mg.

HERBED GREEN BEANS WITH TOMATOES
Recipe 30   *Number of servings:* 4

2 cups   green beans (½ lb. fresh or 1 10-oz. pkg.
          frozen)
  ½   onion, sliced
  1   garlic clove, minced, or 1 tsp. prechopped
         garlic
½ cup   sliced mushrooms
  1   large tomato, cut into thin wedges
1 tsp.   basil
½ tsp.   oregano

1. Steam fresh green beans until slightly crunchy; follow package directions for frozen beans. When done, rinse in cold water to stop cooking. Set aside.
2. While green beans are cooking, spray nonstick skillet with cooking spray. Sauté onion and garlic until tender, stirring frequently. Add small amount of water to prevent sticking.
3. Add mushrooms, tomatoes, basil, and oregano to onions. Stir to prevent sticking. Cook until mushrooms are tender.
4. Add cooked green beans. Stir. Transfer to serving bowl.

NUTRITIONAL SCORECARD
Calories per serving: 41

NUTRIENT	Carbohydrate	Fat	Total Protein	Animal Protein	Sodium
PERCENT CALORIES	78%	6%	16%	0%	
AMOUNT	8.8 G	.3 G	1.8 G	0	6 mg.

SWEET AND SOUR CABBAGE
Recipe 31

Number of servings: 8

1	garlic clove, minced
½ cup	chopped onions
½ cup	raisins
1	apple, grated
8 cups	fine-sliced red cabbage
2 Tbsp.	whole-wheat flour
3 oz.	cider vinegar
2 Tbsp.	fruit concentrate (Mystic Lake Dairy* or apple concentrate)
1 cup	Vecon vegetable broth or defatted chicken broth

1. Spray nonstick skillet with cooking spray. Sauté garlic and onions until onions are translucent. Add small amounts of water to prevent sticking.
2. Combine fruit concentrate, broth, and flour. Add to skillet.
3. Add cabbage, apple, and raisins to skillet. Simmer, covered, until cabbage is tender.

*See shopping list in the beginning of this chapter.

NUTRITIONAL SCORECARD					
Calories per serving: 79					
NUTRIENT	Carbohydrate	Fat	Total Protein	Animal Protein	Sodium
PERCENT CALORIES	88%	3%	9%	0	
AMOUNT	19.3 G	.3 G	1.9 G	0 G	39 mg.

MIX-AND-MATCH VEGETABLES AND SAUCE
Recipe 32   *Number of servings:* 3

10-oz. pkg.   fordhook limas or other vegetable of your
              choice
1 recipe   Sweet Tomato Basil Sauce (recipe #40) or
              other sauce of your choice (recipes #35,
              39–42)

1. Prepare lima beans or other vegetable according to directions on
   package. Do not add salt.
2. Prepare sauce according to recipe. Pour souce over vegetables and
   serve hot.

NUTRITIONAL SCORECARD					
Calories per serving: 97					
NUTRIENT	Carbohydrate	Fat	Total Protein	Animal Protein	Sodium
PERCENT CALORIES	73%	5%	22%	0.	
AMOUNT	18.6 G	.6 G	5.4 G	0 G	100 mg.

LUNCHEON SALAD WITH PESTO SAUCE
Recipe 33   *Number of servings:* 1

1 tomato, sliced
6 slices   cucumber
1 Tbsp.   Pesto Sauce (See recipe #35.)

1. Slice tomato the way you like it. Surround with cucumber slices and
   top with Pesto Sauce.

NUTRITIONAL SCORECARD					
Calories per serving: 51					
NUTRIENT	Carbohydrate	Fat	Total Protein	Animal Protein	Sodium
PERCENT CALORIES	70%	18%	12%	5%	
AMOUNT	9 G	1 G	1.6 G	.67 G	19 mg.

CHEF'S SALAD
Recipe 34

Number of servings: 6

1 head	romaine, Boston, or bibb lettuce (not iceberg)
6	scallions, chopped (white and green parts)
4	radishes, thinly sliced
1	cucumber, thinly sliced
1	broccoli spear, chopped
1 cup	grated carrots
2 stalks	celery, chopped
¼ cup	chopped mushrooms
1	green, red, or yellow bell pepper, sliced

1. Toss ingredients together in a bowl. Your salad will stay crisp for several days if you use a salad spinner.

NUTRITIONAL SCORECARD					
Calories per serving: 29					
NUTRIENT	Carbohydrate	Fat	Total Protein	Animal Protein	Sodium
PERCENT CALORIES	74%	7%	19%	0	
AMOUNT	6.1 G	.3 G	1.5 G	0 G	28 mg.

PESTO SAUCE
Recipe 35

Number of servings: 4

This sauce by itself has a high fat content but, when combined with vegetables, such as the luncheon salad (recipe #33), makes a very acceptable and very delicious dressing. Use fresh herbs. This recipe makes just enough for one vegetable dish.

2 Tbsp.	fresh basil
1 Tbsp.	fresh oregano
2 Tbsp.	fresh parsley
2	cloves garlic, minced
½ tsp.	olive oil
1 tsp.	Parmesan cheese, grated
⅛ tsp.	black pepper

1. Mince all herbs by hand and blend with oil, cheese, and pepper.

NUTRITIONAL SCORECARD
Calories per serving: 21

NUTRIENT	Carbohydrate	Fat	Total Protein	Animal Protein	Sodium
PERCENT CALORIES	51%	38%	11%	3%	
AMOUNT	3 G	1 G	.61 G	.17 G	9 mg.

SPICY SANDWICH SPREAD OR VEGETABLE DIP
Recipe 36   *Number of servings:*

Makes 8–10 sandwiches or 2¼ cups of dip.

This sandwich spread or vegetable dip takes only minutes to make and can be stored in a covered container for four to five days. Try it with raw veggies as a snack when you come home from work. Delicious!

¼	green or red bell pepper
4	radishes
1	small carrot
1	garlic clove
¼	onion
3 sprigs	fresh parsley or ½ tsp. dried
1 cup	garbanzo beans (chickpeas), cooked and drained (If you buy canned beans, rinse well to remove salt.)
¾ cup	low-fat cottage cheese (2%)
1 tsp.	mustard of your choice

1. Combine the bell pepper, radish, carrot, garlic, onion, and parsley in blender. Chop in fine pieces.
2. Add garbanzo beans, cottage cheese, and mustard and blend to desired consistency.

NUTRITIONAL SCORECARD					
Calories per serving: 49					
NUTRIENT	Carbohydrate	Fat	Total Protein	Animal Protein	Sodium
PERCENT CALORIES	53%	14%	33%	19%	
AMOUNT	6.5 G	.8 G	4 G	2.33 G	80 mg.

HEALTHY SOUR CREAM
Recipe 37   *Number of servings:* 8 (2 Tbsp. each serving)

    ½ cup   plain low-fat cottage cheese
    ½ cup   nonfat yogurt
    ½–1 tsp. lemon juice

1. Put all ingredients into the blender and whip until creamy.
2. Mix with Gourmet Sprinkle* or Salsa for a delicious dip or topping for your baked potato.

*See shopping list in the beginning of this chapter.

NUTRITIONAL SCORECARD					
Calories per serving: 21					
NUTRIENT	Carbohydrate	Fat	Total Protein	Animal Protein	Sodium
PERCENT CALORIES	33%	12%	55%	55%	
AMOUNT	1.6 G	.3 G	2.8 G	2.8 G	68 mg.

RASPBERRY VINAIGRETTE DRESSING
Recipe 38   *Number of servings:* 8

A sweet yet tangy salad dressing that will delight your taste buds. Keep it stored in a covered container in the refrigerator for four to five days.

    1½ cups   fresh or frozen raspberries (no sugar added)
    1 cup   cider vinegar
    ¼ cup   fruit concentrate (Mystic Lake Dairy or
                  apple concentrate)
    1½ Tbsp.   cornstarch, dissolved in 3 Tbsp. water

1. Combine raspberries and vinegar in pot and bring to a boil.
2. Remove mixture from heat and strain through a fine sieve to remove raspberry seeds.
3. Return to pot. Add fruit concentrate and return to a boil.
4. Add cornstarch and water mixture to pot, stirring constantly until thickened.
5. Remove from heat. Store in container in refrigerator.

NUTRITIONAL SCORECARD					
Calories per serving: 38					
NUTRIENT	Carbohydrate	Fat	Total Protein	Animal Protein	Sodium
PERCENT CALORIES	94%	4%	2%	0	
AMOUNT	10.8 G	.2 G	.3 G	0 G	0

CREAMY DILL DRESSING
Recipe 39

Number of servings: 2

2 oz.	nonfat yogurt
¼ cup	lemon juice
¼ tsp.	black pepper
½ tsp.	Dijon mustard
2 Tbsp.	fresh dill, minced, or 2 tsp. dried

1. Mix all ingredients. Store in a covered container in refrigerator.

NUTRITIONAL SCORECARD					
Calories per serving: 25					
NUTRIENT	Carbohydrate	Fat	Total Protein	Animal Protein	Sodium
PERCENT CALORIES	70%	4%	26%	25%	
AMOUNT	4.9 G	.1 G	1.8 G	1.6 G	38 mg.

SWEET TOMATO BASIL SAUCE
Recipe 40

Number of servings: 4

This is excellent for fish and all greens.

1½	fresh tomatoes, chopped with ¼ cup water, or 1 tomato from can of tomatoes, crushed
1 Tbsp.	dried basil
1½ tsp.	fruit concentrate (Mystic Lake Dairy or apple concentrate*)

1. Put all ingredients in small skillet. Sauté. Serve over vegetables of your choice.

*See shopping list in the beginning of this chapter.

NUTRITIONAL SCORECARD					
Calories per serving: 18					
NUTRIENT	Carbohydrate	Fat	Total Protein	Animal Protein	Sodium
PERCENT CALORIES	82%	6%	12%	0	
AMOUNT	3.8 G	.1 G	.54 G	0 G	4 mg.

TANGY MUSTARD SAUCE
Recipe 41

Number of servings: 4

This is an excellent sauce for fish and vegetables such as carrots, snow peas, cauliflower, and broccoli.

2 Tbsp.	mustard of your choice
1 tsp.	chopped fresh parsley or ½ tsp. dried
1 Tbsp.	fruit concentrate (Mystic Lake Dairy or apple concentrate*)
1 Tbsp.	orange juice
⅛ tsp.	black pepper

1. Combine all ingredients. Serve over fish or with your favorite vegetable.

*See shopping list in the beginning of this chapter.

NUTRITIONAL SCORECARD
Calories per serving: 20

NUTRIENT	Carbohydrate	Fat	Total Protein	Animal Protein	Sodium
PERCENT CALORIES	69%	21%	10%	0	
AMOUNT	3.4 G	.5 G	.5 G	0 G	98 mg.

LEMONY WINE AND TARRAGON SAUCE
Recipe 42

Number of servings: 4

This is an excellent sauce for fish and carrots.

½ lemon	juiced, or 2 Tbsp. lemon concentrate
½ cup	white wine
1 tsp.	minced fresh tarragon or ⅓ tsp. dried
1 tsp.	chopped fresh parsley or ⅓ tsp. dried
½ tsp.	powdered garlic
½ tsp.	Gourmet Sprinkle* (optional)
⅛ tsp.	black pepper
2 tsp.	cornstarch, dissolved in 1½ Tbsp. water

1. Combine all ingredients in a small saucepan or skillet. Simmer until wine is reduced by one-half.
2. Add cornstarch mixture to pot, and stir constantly over low heat until sauce is thickened.
3. Serve over fish or vegetables of your choice.

*See shopping list in the beginning of this chapter.

NUTRITIONAL SCORECARD					
Calories per serving: 26					
NUTRIENT	Carbohydrate	Fat	Total Protein	Animal Protein	Sodium
PERCENT CALORIES	25%	1%	2%	0	
AMOUNT	1.8 G	.1 G	.13 G	0	2 mg.

*Alcohol contributes 72 percent of the calories.

FRUIT TOPPING
Recipe 43   *Number of servings:* 1

        1   banana
      or
  ½ cup   fresh or frozen berries (strawberries,
              blueberries, or raspberries) or chopped
              peaches or other fruit (without sugar)

1. Peel and core fruit as needed.
2. Puree fruit in blender or food processor to desired consistency, or mash with fork.
3. If fruit is too tart, add Mystic Lake Dairy fruit concentrate or other fruit concentrate as needed.*

*See shopping list in the beginning of this chapter.

NUTRITIONAL SCORECARD

Calories per serving for bananas: 120

NUTRIENT	Carbohydrate	Fat	Total Protein	Animal Protein	Sodium
PERCENT CALORIES	90%	7%	3%	0	
AMOUNT	27 G	1 G	1 G	0	0

Calories per serving for berries: 45–60

NUTRIENT	Carbohydrate	Fat	Total Protein	Animal Protlein	Sodium
PERCENT CALORIES	75–81%	13–17%	6–8%	0	
AMOUNT	10–14 G	1 G	1 G	0	1 mg.

ORANGE SORBET
Recipe 44   *Number of servings:* 4

Actual preparation time is not long, but be sure to add in the freezing time.

1 cup	unsweetened pineapple juice
4	oranges
¼ cup	fruit concentrate (Mystic Lake Dairy; optional)
1 Tbsp.	Triple Sec liqueur (optional)
2 sprigs	fresh mint

1. Cut top off each orange. Scrape out pulp. Keep orange rind "bowls." Deseed orange pulp.
2. Puree deseeded pulp in food processor. Add three-fourths of the pineapple juice. If oranges are tart, add fruit concentrate.
3. Pour liquid into shallow pan and freeze long enough for liquid to harden slightly but not to freeze solid. The time will vary depending on the depth of the freezing pan.
4. When almost frozen, remove and whip in blender. Add the remaining pineapple juice to get creamy consistency. Add Triple Sec at this stage if you want it.
5. Pour liquid into orange shells. Top with fresh mint. Place shells in muffin tray to prevent their rolling over. Freeze again until the consistency of sherbet.

NUTRITIONAL SCORECARD
Calories per serving: 136

NUTRIENT	Carbohydrate	Fat	Total Protein	Animal Protein	Sodium
PERCENT CALORIES	91%	1%	5%	0	
AMOUNT	32.2 G	.2 G	1.7 G	0	1 mg.

*Three percent of the calories come from alcohol.

CALIFORNIA ORBAP COOKIES
Recipe 45

Number of servings: Makes 20 cookies

These cookies get their name from the first letter of the oatmeal, raisins, banana, apple, and peanut butter that are the main ingredients. This recipe makes a spongy, moist cookie.

1 cup	uncooked oatmeal
¼ cup	water
1 cup	raisins
1	green apple, diced with skin
1	banana, pureed
4 Tbsp.	fruit concentrate (Mystic Lake Dairy or apple concentrate*)
4	egg whites
½ cup	whole-wheat pastry or oat flour
2 Tbsp.	natural peanut butter (optional)
½ tsp.	baking soda

1. Moisten the uncooked oatmeal with the water. Add the egg whites and the pureed banana.
2. Mix in the whole-wheat flour and the remaining ingredients.
3. Spray nonstick cookie sheet with cooking spray. Drop 1½-inch to 2-inch cookies on the sheet. Cook at 350° for 12 to 15 minutes. Cookies will be only slightly browned on top, so be careful not to burn the bottoms.

*See shopping list in the beginning of this chapter.

NUTRITIONAL SCORECARD					
Calories per serving: 79					
NUTRIENT	Carbohydrate	Fat	Total Protein	Animal Protein	Sodium
PERCENT CALORIES	76%	14%	10%	2%	
AMOUNT	15.6 G	1.3 G	2.18 G	.3 G	35 mg.

ORANGE BANANA MELANGE
Recipe 46

Number of Servings: 4

This is a very refreshing dessert and takes only ten minutes to prepare. Remember that it will take a couple of hours to set in the refrigerator. You can speed up the process somewhat by using your freezer, but you need to watch it carefully if you do.

2	oranges, peeled and deseeded
2	ripe bananas
1 cup	orange juice
2 envelopes	unflavored gelatin
3 Tbsp.	fruit concentrate (Mystic Lake Dairy or apple concentrate*)

1. Puree oranges, bananas, and fruit concentrate.
2. Bring orange juice to a boil. Sprinkle gelatin into juice. Stir well. Add puree and stir well. Remove from heat. Pour into serving dishes and chill until firm (about 2 to 3 hours).
3. Garnish with fresh mint sprig.

*See shopping list in the beginning of this chapter.

NUTRITIONAL SCORECARD					
Calories per serving: 162					
NUTRIENT	Carbohydrate	Fat	Total Protein	Animal Protein	Sodium
PERCENT CALORIES	86%	3%	11%	7%	
AMOUNT	34.8 G	.6 G	4.6 G	3 G	4 mg.

DANIEL'S JELLY ROLL
Recipe 47   *Number of servings:* 12

7	egg whites
1 cup	whole-wheat pastry flour, sifted
3 Tbsp.	fruit concentrate (Mystic Lake Dairy*)
7 oz.	fruit-only raspberry conserves
1 cup	frozen raspberries, unsweetened
2	bananas

1. Beat egg whites until stiff.
2. Fold egg whites into sifted flour.
3. Put wax paper on cookie sheet with lip, and spray wax paper with Pam. Spread batter onto wax paper–covered cookie sheet. Bake for 6 minutes in preheated oven at 350°.
4. Blend frozen, unsweetened raspberries with raspberry conserves.
5. Take baked dough from cookie sheet (leave wax paper on bottom). Spread raspberry filling evenly over dough. Slice bananas and place on top of filling. Remove wax paper as you roll into a jelly roll. Slice and turn each serving on its side.

*See shopping list in the beginning of this chapter.

NUTRITIONAL SCORECARD					
Calories per serving: 145					
NUTRIENT	Carbohydrate	Fat	Total Protein	Animal Protein	Sodium
PERCENT CALORIES	88%	2%	10%	7%	
AMOUNT	30.4 G	.4 G	3.45 G	2.6 G	45 mg.

BAKED APPLE WITH RAISINS
Recipe 48   *Number of servings:* 1

     1   medium apple
  1 Tbsp. unsulfured raisins
   Dash cinnamon (or to taste)
  1 Tbsp. apple concentrate or Mystic Lake Dairy fruit
          concentrate*

1. Core apple all the way through.
2. Mix raisins, cinnamon, and concentrate together.
3. Put apple in baking dish and fill with mixture.
4. Put ⅛ to ¼ inch of water in baking dish.
5. Cover and cook in microwave for 5 minutes or bake in 400° oven for about 30 minutes, until tender.

*See shopping list in the beginning of this chapter.

NUTRITIONAL SCORECARD					
Calories per serving: 126					
NUTRIENT	Carbohydrate	Fat	Total Protein	Animal Protein	Sodium
PERCENT CALORIES	97%	2%	1%	0	
AMOUNT	33.4 G	.3 G	.4 G	0 G	2 mg.

BAKED BANANA BOAT
Recipe 49   *Number of servings:* 1

    1   medium banana
  1 tsp. fruit-only jam*

1. Do not peel banana. Cut ½ inch off each end.
2. Bake banana for 15 minutes at 350° or until skin turns black (not burned).
3. Using cooking tongs, remove banana, place on plate and slice open lengthwise with a sharp knife. Spoon 1 tsp. of your favorite jam on top and enjoy!

*See shopping list in the beginning of this chapter.

NUTRITIONAL SCORECARD					
Calories per serving: 135					
NUTRIENT	Carbohydrate	Fat	Total Protein	Animal Protein	Sodium
PERCENT CALORIES	90%	7%	3%	0	
AMOUNT	30 G	1 G	1 G	0 G	1 mg.

FRUIT SMOOTHIE
Recipe 50   *Number of servings:* 4

1 cup	orange juice
3 cups	fresh or frozen strawberries
3	ripe bananas
2 Tbsp.	fruit concentrate (Mystic Lake Dairy or apple concentrate*)
10	ice cubes, crushed (approximately 1 cup frozen water)

1. Combine all ingredients in a blender and process until smooth.

*See shopping list in the beginning of this chapter.

NUTRITIONAL SCORECARD
Calories per serving: 173

NUTRIENT	Carbohydrate	Fat	Total Protein	Animal Protein	Sodium
PERCENT CALORIES	87%	8%	5%	0	
AMOUNT	39.1 G	1.6 G	2.1 G	0 G	3 mg.

BAKED RASPBERRY PEAR
Recipe 51   *Number of servings:* 1

1	ripe pear
8	fresh or frozen raspberries
2 Tbsp.	water

1. Cut pear in half and core.
2. Put four berries in each half of the pear. Put pear halves in a covered dish, with 2 tablespoons of water in bottom.
3. Microwave on high until done, about 3 minutes, or bake at 350°.

NUTRITIONAL SCORECARD
Calories per serving: 115

NUTRIENT	Carbohydrate	Fat	Total Protein	Animal Protein	Sodium
PERCENT CALORIES	87%	9%	4%	0	
AMOUNT	28.5 G	1.3 G	1.3 G	0 G	2 mg.

Now That You've Read This Book

This book has given you a four-point program of nutrition, exercise, visualization, and oxygen production to increase your energy and banish tiredness from your life forever. Our final words of advice are these:

- *Start today.* Even if you take only one little step toward the Never Be Tired Again goals today, one little step is better than nothing.

- *Do it for yourself.* You've been taking care of other people all of your adult life. Now it's time to take care of you! Don't do the Never Be Tired Again program for your spouse, for your children, for your business, or for any other reason. Do it for yourself!

- *Don't expect to be perfect.* If you occasionally revert to old, low-energy habits, don't consider yourself a failure. Consider yourself human. Progress is never in a straight line. It's a series of zigzags and plateaus. The real mark of a winner is the ability to pick yourself up, dust yourself off, and keep going.

Once you have attained your energy level and weight and cholesterol goals, allow yourself an occasional change of pace. If you live the Never Be Tired Again program 90 percent of the time, you'll have more energy and better health than you ever dreamed possible!

- *Expect to succeed.* You can do it!

Selected References and Recommended Reading

BARKER, SARAH. *The Alexander Technique*. New York: Bantam Books, 1978.

BENSON, H. "Decreased Alcohol Intake Associated with Practice of Meditation: A Retrospective Investigation." *Annals of the New York Academy of Sciences*, April 1974, 233, 174–177.

BLUME, ELAINE. "Do Artificial Sweeteners Help You Lose Weight?" *Nutrition Action Healthletter*, May 1987, 14(4), 1, 4–5.

——————— "Overdosing on Protein." *Nutriton Action Healthletter*, March 1987, 14(2), 1.

BLUMENTHAL, JAMES A.; WILLIAMS, R. SANDERS; NEEDELS, TERRI L.; and WALLACE, ANDREW G. "Psychological Changes Accompany Aerobic Exercise in Healthy Middle-aged Adults." *Psychosomatic Medicine*, December 1982, 44(6), 529–536.

BONJOUR, J. P. "Biotin in Man's Nutrition and Therapy—a Review." *International Journal of Vitamin and Nutritional Research*, 1977, 47:107.

BORKAN, G. A., and NORRIS, A. H. "Assessment of Biological Age Using a Profile of Physical Parameters." *Journal of Gerontology*, March 1980, 35(2), 177–184.

BROWN, BARBARA B. *Supermind: The Ultimate Energy*. New York: Bantam Books, 1980.

BROWN, DANIEL, *et al.* "Differences in Visual Sensitivity Among Mindfulness Meditators and Non-meditators." *Perceptual and Motor Skills*, June 1984, 58(3), 727–33.

BRUCE, R. A. "Exercise, Functional Aerobic Capacity, and Aging—Another Viewpoint." *Medical Science of Sports Exercise*, 1984, 16(1), 8–13.

CAPRA, FRITJOF. *The Tao of Physics*. New York: Bantam Books, 1977.

CHEN, MARTIN K. (ED). "The Epidemiology of Self-perceived Fatigue Among Adults." *Preventive Medicine*, 1986, Vol. 15, 74–81.

COHEN, LEONARD A. "Diet and cancer." *Scientific American*, November 1987, 257(5), 42–48.

COMBS, G. F., JR.; NOGUCHI, T.; AND SCOTT, M. L. "Mechanisms of Action of Selenium and Vitamin E in Protection of Biological Membranes." *Federation Proceedings*, October 1975, 34(11), 2090–2095.

CONDRA, MICHAEL, et al. "Prevalence and Significance of Tobacco Smoking in Impotence." *Urology*, June 1986, 26(6).

COOPER, KENNETH H. *The Aerobics Program for Total Well-Being*. New York: Bantam Books, 1982.

COOPER, K. H.; POLLOCK, M. L.; MARTIN, R. P.; et al. "Physical Fitness Levels vs. Selected Coronary Risk Factors: A Cross-sectional Study." *Journal of the American Medical Association*, 1976, 236:165–169.

COYLE, EDWARD F.; COGGAN, ANDREW R.; HEMMERT, MARI K.; AND IVY, JOHN L. "Muscle Glycogen Utilization During Prolonged Strenuous Exercise When Fed Carbohydrate." *Journal of Applied Physiology*, July 1986, 61(1), 165–172.

EISENBERG, DAVID, WITH WRIGHT, THOMAS LEE. *Encounters with Qi*. New York: Penguin Books, 1987.

"The Fatigue Virus." University of California, Berkeley, *Wellness Letter*, November 1987, 4(2), 1.

FRANKEL, B. L.; PATEL, D. J.; HORWITZ, D.; FRIEDEWALD, W. T.; AND GAARDER, K. R. "Treatment of Hypertension with Biofeedback and Relaxation Techniques." *Psychosomatic Medicine*, June 1978, 40(4), 276–293.

FUNDERBURK, JAMES. *Science Studies Yoga*. Honesdale, Pennsylvania: The Himalayan International Institute of Yoga Science and Philosophy of USA, 1977.

GARDNER, D. C., AND BEATTY, G. J. "How Fit Are Americans?" Research paper presented at the annual convention of the American Board of Medical Psychotherapists, Cancun, Mexico, May 1987.

———. *Stop Stress and Aging Now*. Windham, New Hampshire: American Training and Research Associates, Inc., 1985.

GAWAIN, SHAKTI. *Creative Visualization*. New York: Bantam Books, 1985.

GENDEL, EVALYN S. "Lack of Fitness a Source of Chronic Ills in Woman." *The Physician and Sportsmedicine*, February 1978, 85–95.

GRIM, PAUL F. "Relaxation Therapies and Neurosis: A Central Fatigue Interpretation." *Psychosomatics*, November/December 1972, 13(6), 363–370.

HAREER, A. F. "Coronary Heart Disease—An Epidemic Related to Diet?" *American Journal of Clinical Nutrition*, April 1983, 37(4), 669–681.

HARMAN, D. "The Aging Process." *Proceedings of the National Academy of Science—U.S.A.*, November 1981, 78(11), 7124–7128.

HARRIS, W. S.; CONNOR, W. E.; AND McMURRY, M. P. "The Comparative Reductions of the Plasma Lipids and Lipo Proteins by Dietary Polyunsaturated Fats: Salmon Oil vs. Vegetable Oils." *Metabolism: Clinical and Experimental*, February 1983, 32(2), 179–184.

HEGSTED, D. M. "Serum-cholesterol Response to Dietary Cholesterol: A Re-evaluation." *American Journal of Clinical Nutrition*, August 1986, 44(2), 299–305.

HEGSTED, D. M. "Dietary Standards—Guidelines for Prevention of Deficiency or Prescription for Total Health?" *Journal of Nutrition*, March 1986, 116(3), 478–481.

HERBERT, NICK. *Quantum Reality.* Garden City, New York: Anchor Books, 1987.

HITTLEMAN, RICHARD L. *Be Young with Yoga.* New York: Paperback Library, Inc., 1962.

HOUSE, JAMES S. *Work Stress and Social Support.* Reading, Massachusetts: Addison-Wesley Publishing Company, 1981.

HOARD, R. B., AND HERBOLD, N. H. *Nutrition in Clinical Care.* New York: McGraw-Hill Book Company, 1982.

HUGHES, JOHN R.; CROW, RICHARD S.; JACOBS, DAVID R., JR.; MITTELMARK, MAURICE B.; AND LEON, ARTHUR S. "Physical Activity, Smoking, and Exercise-Induced Fatigue." *Journal of Behavioral Medicine*, 1984, 7(2), 217–230.

IYENGAR, B. K. S. "Restorative Asanas for a Healthy Immune System." *Yoga Journal*, July/August 1987, 47–49.

JACOBSON, MICHAEL. *Chemical Cuisine.* Washington, D.C.: Center for Science in the Public Interest, 1986.

KAKU, MICHIO, AND TRAINER, JENNIFER. *Beyond Einstein: The Cosmic Quest for the Theory of the Universe.* New York: Bantam Books, 1987.

KATZ, JANE, WITH BRUNING, NANCY P. *Swimming for Total Fitness.* Garden City, New York: Dolphin Books/Doubleday & Company, Inc., 1981.

KAUFMAN, DOUG A., WITH SKOLNIK, RACQUEL. *The Food Sensitivity Diet.* Toronto: PaperJacks Ltd., 1986.

KENDLER, BARRY S. "Garlic *(Allium sativum)* and Onion *(Allium cepa):* A review of Their Relationship to Cardiovascular Disease." *Preventive Medicine*, September, 1987, 16:5, 670–685.

KENT, D. C., AND CENCI, L. "Smoking and the Workplace: Tobacco Smoke Health Hazards to the Involuntary Smoker." *Journal of Medicine*, June 1982, 24(6), 469–472.

KILHMAN, CHRISTOPHER. *The Complete Shoppers' Guide to Natural Foods.* Brookline, Massachusetts: The Autumn Press, 1980.

KONISHI, F., AND HARRISON, S. L. "Vitamin D for Adults." *Journal of Nutrition Education*, 1980, 11:120.

KROHNE, HEINZ W., AND LAUX, LOTHAR (EDS). *Achievement, Stress, and Anxiety.* Washington, D.C.: Hemisphere Publishing Co., 1982.

KUSHI, MICHIO, AND THE EAST WEST FOUNDATION. *The Macrobiotic Ap-*

proach to Cancer. Wayne, New Jersey: Avery Publishing Group, Inc., 1982.

LEFCOURT, HERBERT M. *Locus of Control Current Trends in Theory and Research.* Hillsdale, New Jersey: Lawrence Erlbaum Associates, Publishers, 1976.

LEVINE, AGRAHA. "Limitless Fountain of Energy." *Meditation,* Summer 1987, II(3), 30–33.

LIEBMAN, BONNIE F., AND COLBURN, MARY. *Sodium Scoreboard.* Washington, D.C.: Center for Science in the Public Interest, 1982.

LIEBMAN, BONNIE F., AND JACOBSON, MICHAEL. *CSPI's Anti-Cancer Eating Guide.* Washington, D.C.: Center for Science in the Public Interest, 1984.

——————.*CSPI's Sugar Scoreboard.* Washington, D.C.: Center for Science in the Public Interest, 1985.

MASTERS, WILLIAM H. "Sex and Aging—Expectations and Reality." *Hospital Practice,* August, 1986, 21:8, 175–198.

MONTGOMERY, GEORGE K. "Uncommon Tiredness Among College Undergraduates." *Journal of Consulting and Clinical Psychology,* 1983, 51(4), 517–525.

NATIONAL ACADEMY OF SCIENCES FOOD AND NUTRITION BOARD. *Recommended Dietary Allowances,* rev. 9th ed. Washington, D.C., National Academy of Sciences, 1980.

NUERNBERGER, PHIL. *Freedom from Stress.* Honesdale, Pennsylvania: Himalayan International Institute of Yoga, Science and Philosophy, 1981.

ORNISH, DEAN. *Stress, Diet and Your Heart.* New York: Holt, Rinehart and Winston, 1982.

PAFFENBARGER, R. S., AND HYDE, R. T. "Exercise in the Prevention of Coronary Heart Disease." *Preview of Medicine,* January 1984, 13(1), 3–22.

PALMER, S. "Diet, Nutrition, and Cancer: The Future of Dietary Policy. *Cancer Research,* May 1983, 43(suppl.), 2509s–2514s.

PATEL, C. H. "Biofeedback-Aided Relaxation and Meditation in the Management of Hypertension." *Biofeedback Self Regulation,* March 1977, 2(1), 1–41.

——————. "Yoga and Bio-feedback in the Management of Hypertension." *Lancet,* November 1973, 2(837), 1053–1055.

PAULING, LINUS. *How to Live Longer and Feel Better.* New York: Avon Books, 1987.

PETERSON, C., AND SELIGMAN, M. E. "Explanatory Style and Illness." *Journal of Personality,* June, 1987, 55(2), 237–265.

PORTA, F. A.; JOWN, N. S.; AND NITTA, R. T. "Effects of the Type of Dietary Fat at Two Levels of Vitamin E in Wistar Male Rats During Development and Aging: I. Life Span, Serum Biochemical Parameters and Pathological Change. *Mechanisms of Aging and Development,* May 1980, 13(1), 1–39.

RAMA, SWAMI; BALLENTINE, RUDOLPH; AND HYMES, ALAN. *Science of Breath.* Honesdale, Pennsylvania: The Himalayan International Institute of Yoga Science and Philosophy, 1979.

ROBERTSON, J.; BRYDON, W. G.; TADESSE, G.; WENHAM, P.; WALLS, A.; AND EASTWOOD, M. A. "The Effect of Raw Carrot on Serum Lipids and Colon Function." *American Journal of Clinical Nutrition,* September 1979, 32(9), 1889–1992.

ROCKWELL, DON A., AND BURR, BILL D. "The Tired Patient." *The Journal of Family Practice,* 1977, 5(5), 853–857.

ROSENTHAL, NORMAN E.; GENHART, MICHAEL; JACOBSEN, FREDERICK M.; SKWERER, ROBERT G.; AND WEHR, THOMAS A. "Disturbances of Appetite and Weight Regulation in Seasonal Affective disorder." *Annals of the New York Academy of Sciences,* 1987, 499:216–230.

ROTTER, J. B. "Generalized Expectancies for Internal versus External Control of Reinforcement." *Psychological Monographs,* 80(1, whole No. 609), 1, 966.

SCHATZ, MARY PULLIG. "Yoga, the Mind, and Immunity." *Yoga Journal,* July/August 1987, 42–46.

SCHORIN, MARILYN D. "Nutrition, Physical Fitness, and Athletic Performance." In: *Nutrition in Clinical Care,* (Howard, R. B., and Herbold, N. H., eds.) New York: McGraw-Hill Book Co., 1982, 191–209.

SCHULLER, ROBERT H. *Tough Times Never Last, but Tough People Do!* New York: Bantam Books, 1983.

SHERWOOD, KEITH. *The Art of Spiritual Healing.* St. Paul, Minnesota: Llewellyn Publications, 1986.

SHIMONY, ABNER. "The Reality of the Quantum World." *Scientific American,* January 1988, 258(1), 46–53.

Shopper's Guide to Natural Foods, by the editors of the East West Journal. Garden City Park, New York: Avery Publishing Group, Inc. 1987.

SHUBIK, P. "Potential Carcinogenicity of Food Additives and Contaminants." *Cancer Research,* November 1975, 35 (11 Part 2), 3475–3480.

SILVER, NAN. "Do Optimists Live Longer?" *American Health,* November 1986, 50–53.

SOLBERG, LEIF I. "Lassitude." *Journal of the American Medical Association,* 1984, 251(24), 3272–3276.

SPRING, B.; MALLER, O.; WURTMAN, J.; DIGMAN, L.; COZOLINO, L. "Effects of Protein and Carbohydrate Meals on Mood and Performance: Interactions with Sex and Age." *Journal of Psychological Research,* 1982–83, 17(2), 155–167.

STAMFORD, BRYANT. "Does Lactic Acid Cause Muscle Fatigue?" *The Physician and Sportsmedicine,* June 1985, 13(6), 193.

STAPP, H. "The Copenhagen Interpretation and the Nature of Spacetime. *American Journal of Physics,* 40, 1972, 1098.

STORMAN, MARTIN D. "Marital Satisfaction Variables and Female Breast Cancer Patients' Predictions of Their Life Expectancies." *Dissertation Abstracts International,* July 1982, 43(1-B), 266.

STOYVA, JOHANN (ed.). *Biofeedback and Self-Regulation.* New York: Plenum Publishing, 1980.

STUNKARD, A. J. "Nutrition, Aging and Obesity: A Critical Review of a Complex Relationship." *International Journal of Obesity,* 1983, 7(3), 201–220.

THAYER, ROBERT E. "Energy, Tiredness, and Tension Effects of a Sugar Snack Versus Moderate Exercise." *Journal of Personality and Social Psychology,* 1987 52(1), 119–125.

TOBEN, BOB, AND WOLF, FRED ALAN. *Space-Time and Beyond.* New York: Bantam Books, 1987.

U.S. DEPARTMENT OF AGRICULTURE. "The Sodium Content of Your Food." Home and Garden bulletin number 233.

VIRAG, R.; BOUILLY, P.; FRYDMAN, D. "Is Impotence an Arterial Disorder?" *The Lancet,* January, 1985, 8422, 181–184.

WALDRON, I. "Sex Differences in Human Mortality: The Role of Genetic Factors." *Society of Science Medicine,* 1983, 17(6), 321–333.

WALFORD, R. L. "Immunologic Theory of Aging: Current Status." *Federation Proceedings,* Setpember 1974, 33(9), 2020–2027.

WEBER, F.; BERNARD, R. J.; AND ROY, D. "Effects of High-Complex-Carbohydrate, Low-Fat Diet and Daily Exercise on Individuals 70 Years of Age and Older. *Journal of Gerontology,* March 1983, 38(2), 155–161.

WEHR, THOMAS A.; SKWERER, ROBERT G.; JACOBSEN, FREDERICK M.; SACK, DAVID A.; AND ROSENTHAL, NORMAN E. "Eye versus Skin Phototherapy of Seasonal Affective Disorder. *American Journal of Psychiatry,* June 1987, 144(6), 753–757.

WILLIAMS, CLYDE. "Nutritional Aspects of Exercise-Induced Fatigue." *Proceedings of the Nutrition Society,* 1985, 44:245–256.

WOLF, FRED ALAN. *The Body Quantum.* New York: MacMillan Publishing Co., 1986.

——————. *Taking the Quantum Leap.* San Francisco, California: Harper & Row, 1981.

WOOD, REBECCA. "Ranking the Sweeteners." *Bestways,* December 1987, 28–29.

WOZNIAK, DAVID F.; FINGER, STANLEY; BLUMENTHAL, HERMAN; POLAND, RUSSELL F. "Brain Damage, Stress, and Life Span: An Experimental Study." *Journal of Gerontology,* March 1982, 37(2), 161–168.

WURTMAN, J. J. *Managing Your Mind and Mood Through Food.* New York: Rawson Associates, 1986.

WURTMAN, R. J., AND WURTMAN, J. J. "Nutrients, Neurotransmitter Synthesis, and the Control of Food Intake." *Res. Pub. Assoc. Res. Nerv. Mental Disorders,* 1984, 62, 77–86.

YOUNG, E. A. "Nutrition, Aging and the Aged." *Medical Clinics of North America,* March 1983, 67(2), 295–313.

ZUKAV, GARY. *The Dancing Wu Li Masters.* New York: Bantam Books, 1979.

OUR "PERSONAL FAVORITES" LIST OF HEALTH-ORIENTED MAGAZINES AND NEWSLETTERS

American Health. 80 Fifth Avenue, New York, NY 10011; $1.95 per issue, $14.95 per 10-issue subscription rate.

Bestways, P.O. Box 2028, Carson City, NV 89702; $1.95 per issue, $18.00 per year subcription rate.

EastWest Journal, 17 Station Street, Box 1200, Brookline, MA 02147; $2.00 per issue, $18 per year subscription rate.

Lowfat Lifeline, 52 Condolea Court, Lake Oswego, OR 97035; $15 per year subscription rate.

Nutrition Action Health Letter, published by the Center for Science in the Public Interest, 1501 16th Street, NW, Washington, DC 20036; $19.95 for 10 issues per year and membership in the organization. All but $5 of the membership fee—which pays for the subscription—is tax-deductible.

Prevention, 33 East Minor Street, Emmaus, PA 18098; $1.50 per issue, $13.97 per year subscription rate.

University of California, Berkeley Wellness Letter, P.O. Box 10922, Des Moines, IA 50340; $20 per year subscription rate.

Vegetarian Times, P.O. Box 570, Oak Park, IL 60303; $2.50 per copy, $24.95 per year subscription rate.

Yoga Journal, P.O. Box 6076, Syracuse, NY 13217; $3.00 per issue, $15.00 subscription rate.

Index